OF THE EPIDEMICS

Hippocrates of Kos
Father of Medicine

Translated: Francis Adams
Edited by: D.P. Curtin

Dalcassian
Publishing
Company

PHILADELPHIA, PA

Letter to the Themistius the Philosopher

Library of Congress Cataloging-in-Publication Data

Book One

Section One

1. In Thasus, about the autumn equinox, and under the Pleiades, the rains were abundant, constant, and soft, with southerly winds; the winter southerly, the northerly winds faint, droughts; on the whole, the winter having the character of spring. The spring was southerly, cool, rains small in quantity. Summer, for the most part, cloudy, no rain, the Etesian winds, rare and small, blew in an irregular manner. The whole constitution of the season being thus inclined to the southerly, and with droughts early in the spring, from the preceding opposite and northerly state, ardent fevers occurred in a few instances, and these very mild, being rarely attended with hemorrhage, and never proving fatal. Swellings appeared about the ears, in many on either side, and in the greatest number on both sides, being unaccompanied by fever so as not to confine the patient to bed; in all cases they disappeared without giving trouble, neither did any of them come to suppuration, as is common in swellings from other causes. They were of a lax, large, diffused character, without inflammation or pain, and they went away without any critical sign. They seized children, adults, and mostly those who were engaged in the exercises of the palestra and gymnasium, but seldom attacked women. Many had dry coughs without expectoration, and accompanied with hoarseness of voice. In some instances earlier, and in others later, inflammations with pain seized sometimes one of the testicles, and sometimes both; some of these cases were accompanied with fever and some not; the greater part of these were attended with much suffering. In other respects they were free of disease, so as not to require medical assistance.

2. Early in the beginning of spring, and through the summer, and towards winter, many of those who had been long gradually declining, took to bed with symptoms of phthisis; in many cases formerly of a doubtful character the disease then became confirmed; in these the constitution inclined to the phthisical. Many, and, in fact, the most of them, died; and of those confined to bed, I do not know if a single individual survived for any considerable time; they died more suddenly than is common in such cases. But other diseases, of a protracted character, and attended with fever, were well supported, and did not prove fatal: of these we will give a description afterwards.

Consumption was the most considerable of the diseases which then prevailed, and the only one which proved fatal to many persons. Most of them were affected by these diseases in the following manner: fevers accompanied with rigors, of the continual type, acute, having no complete intermissions, but of the form of the semi-tertians, being milder the one day, and the next having an exacerbation, and increasing in violence; constant sweats, but not diffused over the whole body; extremities very cold, and warmed with difficulty; bowels disordered, with bilious, scanty, unmixed, thin, pungent, and frequent dejections. The urine was thin, colorless, unconcocted, or thick, with a deficient sediment, not settling favorably, but casting down a crude and unseasonable sediment. Sputa small, dense, concocted, but brought up rarely and with difficulty; and in those who encountered the most violent symptoms there was no concoction at all, but they continued throughout spitting crude matters. Their fauces, in most of them, were painful from first to last, having redness with inflammation; defluxions thin, small and acrid; they were soon wasted and became worse, having no appetite for any kind of food throughout; no thirst; most persons delirious when near death. So much concerning the phthisical affections.

3. In the course of the summer and autumn many fevers of the continual type, but not violent; they attacked persons who had been long indisposed, but who were otherwise not in an uncomfortable state. In most cases the bowels were disordered in a very moderate degree, and they did not suffer thereby in any manner worth mentioning; the urine was generally well colored, clear, thin, and after a time becoming concocted near the crisis. They had not much cough, nor it troublesome; they were not in appetite, for it was necessary to give them food (on the whole, persons laboring under phthisis were not affected in the usual manner). They were affected with fevers, rigors, and deficient sweats, with varied and irregular paroxysms, in general not intermitting, but having exacerbations in the tertian form. The earliest crisis which occurred was about the twentieth day, in most about the fortieth, and in many about the eighteenth. But there were cases in which it did not leave them thus at all, but in an irregular manner, and without any crisis; in most of these the fevers, after a brief interval, relapsed again; and from these relapses they came to a crisis in the same periods; but in many they were prolonged so that the disease was not gone at the approach of winter. Of all those which are

described under this constitution, the phthisical diseases alone were of a fatal character; for in all the others the patients bore up well, and did not die of the other fevers.

Section Two

1. In Thasus, early in autumn, the winter suddenly set in rainy before the usual time, with much northerly and southerly winds. These things all continued so during the season of the Pleiades, and until their setting. The winter was northerly, the rains frequent, in torrents, and large, with snow, but with a frequent mixture of fair weather. These things were all so, but the setting in of the cold was not much out of season. After the winter solstice, and at the time when the zephyr usually begins to blow, severe winterly storms out of season, with much northerly wind, snow, continued and copious rains; the sky tempestuous and clouded; these things were protracted, and did not remit until the equinox. The spring was cold, northerly, rainy, and clouded; the summer was not very sultry, the Etesian winds blew constant, but quickly afterwards, about the rising of Arcturus, there were again many rains with north winds. The whole season being wet, cold, and northerly, people were, for the most part, healthy during winter; but early in the spring very many, indeed, the greater part, were valetudinary. At first ophthalmies set in, with rheums, pains, unconcocted discharges, small concretions, generally breaking with difficulty, in most instances they relapsed, and they did not cease until late in autumn. During summer and autumn there were dysenteric affections, attacks of tenesmus and lientery, bilious diarrhoea, with thin, copious, undigested, and acrid dejections, and sometimes with watery stools; many had copious defluxions, with pain, of a bilious, watery, slimy, purulent nature, attended with strangury, not connected with disease of the kidneys, but one complaint succeeding the other; vomitings of bile, phlegm, and undigested food, sweats, in all cases a redundance of humors. In many instances these complaints were unattended with fever, and did not prevent the patients from walking about, but some cases were febrile, as will be described. In some all those described below occurred with pain. During autumn, and at the commencement of winter, there were phthisical complaints, continual fevers; and, in a few cases, ardent; some diurnal, others nocturnal, semi-tertians, true tertians, quartans, irregular fevers.

2. All these fevers described attacked great numbers. All these fevers attacked the smallest numbers, and the patients suffered the least from them, for there were no hemorrhages, except a few and to a small amount, nor was there delirium; all the other complaints were slight; in these the crises were regular, in most instances, with the intermittents, in seventeen days; and I know no instance of a person dying of causus, nor becoming phrenitic. The tertians were more numerous than the ardent fevers, and attended with more pain; but these all had four periods in regular succession from the first attack, and they had a complete crisis in seven, without a relapse in any instance. The quartans attacked many at first, in the form of regular quartans, but in no few cases a transition from other fevers and diseases into quartans took place; they were protracted, as is wont with them, indeed, more so than usual. Quotidian, nocturnal, and wandering fevers attacked many persons, some of whom continued to keep up, and others were confined to bed. In most instances these fevers were prolonged under the Pleiades and till winter. Many persons, and more especially children, had convulsions from the commencement; and they had fever, and the convulsions supervened upon the fevers; in most cases they were protracted, but free from danger, unless in those who were in a deadly state from other complaints. Those fevers which were continual in the main, and with no intermissions, but having exacerbations in the tertian form, there being remissions the one day and exacerbations the next, were the most violent of all those which occurred at that time, and the most protracted, and occurring with the greatest pains, beginning mildly, always on the whole increasing, and being exacerbated, and always turning worse, having small remissions, and after an abatement having more violent paroxysms, and growing worse, for the most part, on the critical days. Rigors, in all cases, took place in an irregular and uncertain manner, very rare and weak in them, but greater in all other fevers; frequent sweats, but most seldom in them, bringing no alleviation, but, on the contrary, doing mischief. Much cold of the extremities in them, and these were warmed with difficulty. Insomnolency, for the most part, especially in these fevers, and again a disposition to coma. The bowels, in all diseases, were disordered, and in a bad state, but worst of all in these. The urine, in most of them, was either thin and crude, yellow, and after a time with slight symptoms of concoction in a critical form, or having the proper thickness, but muddy, and neither settling nor subsiding; or having small and bad, and crude sediments; these being the worst of all.

Coughs attended these fevers, but I cannot state that any harm or good ever resulted from the cough.

3. The most of these were protracted and troublesome, went on in a very disorderly and irregular form, and, for the most part, did in a crisis, either in the fatal cases or in the others; for if it left some of them for a season it soon returned again. In a few instances the lever terminated with a crisis; in the earliest of these about the eightieth day, and some of these relapsed, so that most of them were not free from the fever during the winter; but the fever left most of them without a crisis, and these things happened alike to those who recovered and to those who did not. There being much want of crisis and much variety as to these diseases, the greatest and worst symptom attended the most of them, namely, a loathing of all articles of food, more especially with those who had otherwise fatal symptoms; but they were not unseasonably thirsty in such fevers. After a length of time, with much suffering and great wasting, abscesses were formed in these cases, either unusually large, so that the patients could not support them, or unusually small, so that they did no good, but soon relapsed and speedily got worse. The diseases which attacked them were in the form of dysenteries, tenesmus, lientery, and fluxes; but, in some cases, there were dropsies, with or without these complaints. Whatever attacked them violently speedily cut them off, or again, did them no good. Small rashes, and not corresponding to the violence of the disease, and quickly disappearing, or swellings occurred about the ears, which were not resolved, and brought on no crisis. In some they were determined to the joints, and especially to the hip-joint, terminating critically with a few, and quickly again increasing to its original habit.

4. People died of all these diseases, but mostly of these fevers, and notably infants just weaned, and older children, until eight or ten years of age, and those before puberty. These things occurred to those affected with the complaints described above, and to many persons at first without them. The only favorable symptom, and the greatest of those which occurred, and what saved most of those who were in the greatest dangers, was the conversion of it to a strangury, and when, in addition to this, abscesses were formed. The strangury attacked, most especially, persons of the ages I have mentioned, but it also occurred in many others, both of those who were not confined to bed and those who were. There was a speedy and great change in all these cases. For

the bowels, if they happened previously to have watery discharges of a bad character, became regular, they got an appetite for food, and the fevers were mild afterwards. But, with regard to the strangury itself, the symptoms were protracted and painful. Their urine was copious, thick, of various characters, red, mixed with pus, and was passed with pain. These all recovered, and I did not see a single instance of death among them. 5. With regard to the dangers of these cases, one must always attend to the seasonable concoction of all the evacuations, and to the favorable and critical abscesses. The concoctions indicate a speedy crisis and recovery of health; crude and undigested evacuations, and those which are converted into bad abscesses, indicate either want of crisis, or pains, or prolongation of the disease, or death, or relapses; which of these it is to be must be determined from other circumstances. The physician must be able to tell the antecedents, know the present, and foretell the future- must mediate these things, and have two special objects in view with regard to disease, namely, to do good or to do no harm. The art consists in three things-the disease, the patient, and the physician. The physician is the servant of the art, and the patient must combat the disease along with the physician.

6. Pains about the head and neck, and heaviness of the same along with pain, occur either without fevers or in fevers. Convulsions occurring in persons attacked with frenzy, and having vomitings of verdigris-green bile, in some cases quickly prove fatal. In ardent fevers, and in those other fevers in which there is pain of the neck, heaviness of the temples, mistiness about the eyes, and distention about the hypochondriac region, not unattended with pain, hemorrhage from the nose takes place, but those who have heaviness of the whole head, cardialgia and nausea, vomit bilious and pituitous matters; children, in such affections, are generally attacked with convulsions, and women have these and also pains of the uterus; whereas, in elder persons, and those in whom the heat is already more subdued, these cases end in paralysis, mania, and loss of sight.

Section Three

7. In Thasus, a little before and during the season of Arcturus, there were frequent and great rains, with northerly winds. About the equinox, and till the setting of the Pleiades, there were a few southerly rains: the winter northerly and parched, cold, with great winds and

snow. Great storms about the equinox, the spring northerly, dryness, rains few and cold. About the summer solstice, scanty rains, and great cold until near the season of the Dog-star. After the Dog-days, until the season of Arcturus, the summer hot, great droughts, not in intervals, but continued and severe: no rain; the Etesian winds blew; about the season of Arcturus southerly rains until the equinox.

8. In this state of things, during winter, paraplegia set in, and attacked many, and some died speedily; and otherwise the disease prevailed much in an epidemical form, but persons remained free from all other diseases. Early in the spring, ardent fevers commenced and continued through the summer until the equinox. Those then that were attacked immediately after the commencement of the spring and summer, for the most part recovered, and but few of them died. But when the autumn and the rains had set in, they were of a fatal character, and the greater part then died. When in these attacks of ardent fevers there was a proper and copious hemorrhage from the nose, they were generally saved by it, and I do not know a single person who had a proper hemorrhage who died in this constitution. Philiscus, Epaminon, and Silenus, indeed, who had a trifling epistaxis on the fourth and fifth day, died. Most of those taken with had a rigor about the time of the crisis, and notably those who had no hemorrhage; these had also rigor associated.

9. Some were attacked with jaundice on the sixth day, but these were benefited either by an urinary purgation, or a disorder of the bowels, or a copious hemorrhage, as in the case of Heraclides, who was lodged with Aristocydes: this person, though he had the hemorrhage from the nose, the purgation by the bladder, and disorder of the bowels, experienced a favorable crisis on the twentieth day, not like the servant of Phanagoras, who had none of these symptoms, and died. The hemorrhages attacked most persons, but especially young persons and those in the prime of life, and the greater part of those who had not the hemorrhage died: elderly persons had jaundice or disorder of the bowels, such as Bion, who was lodged with Silenus. Dysenteries were epidemical during the summer, and some of those cases in which the hemorrhage occurred, terminated in dysentery, as happened to the slave of Eraton, and to Mullus, who had a copious hemorrhage, which settled down into dysentery, and they recovered. This humor was redundant in many cases, since in those who had not the hemorrhage

about the crisis, but the risings about the ears disappeared, after their disappearance there was a sense of weight in the left flank extending to the extremity of the hip, and pain setting in after the crisis, with a discharge of thin urine; they began to have small hemorrhages about the twenty-fourth day, and the swelling was converted into the hemorrhage. In the case of Antiphon, the son of Critobulus' son, the fever ceased and came to a crisis about the fortieth day.

10. Many women were seized, but fewer than of the men, and there were fewer deaths among them. But most of them had difficult parturition, and after labor they were taken ill, and these most especially died, as, for example, the daughter of Telebolus died on the sixth day after delivery. Most females had the menstrual discharge during the fever, and many girls had it then for the first time: in certain individuals both the hemorrhage from the nose and the menses appeared; thus, in the case of the virgin daughter of Daetharses, the menses then took place for the first time, and she had also a copinous hemorrhage from the nose, and I knew no instance of any one dying when one or other of these took place properly. But all those in the pregnant state that were attacked had abortions, as far as I observed. The urine in most cases was of the proper color, but thin, and having scanty sediments: in most the bowels were disordered with thin and bilious dejections; and many, after passing through the other crises, terminated in dysenteries, as happened to Xenophanes and Critias. The urine was watery, copious, clear, and thin; and even after the crises, when the sediment was natural, and all the other critical symptoms were favorable, as I recollect having happened to Bion, who was lodged in the house of Silenus, and Critias, who lived with Xenophanes, the slave of Areton, and the wife of Mnesistratus. But afterwards all these were attacked with dysentery. It would be worth while to inquire whether the watery urine was the cause of this. About the season of Arcturus many had the crisis on the eleventh day, and in them the regular relapses did not take place, but they became comatose about this time, especially children; but there were fewest deaths of all among them.

11. About the equinox, and until the season of the Pleiades, and at the approach of winter, many ardent fevers set in; but great numbers at that season were seized with phrenitis, and many died; a few cases also occurred during the summer. These then made their attack at the

commencement of ardent fevers, which were attended with fatal symptoms; for immediately upon their setting in, there were acute fever and small rigors, insomnolency, aberration, thirst, nausea, insignificant sweats about the forehead and clavicles, but no general perspiration; they had much delirious talking, fears, despondency, great coldness of the extremities, in the feet, but more especially in their hands: the paroxysms were on the even days; and in most cases, on the fourth day, the most violent pains set in, with sweats, generally coldish, and the extremities could not be warmed, but were livid and rather cold, and they had then no thirst; in them the urine was black, scanty, thin, and the bowels were constipated; there was an hemorrhage from the nose in no case in which these symptoms occurred, but merely a trifling epistaxis; and none of them had a relapse, but they died on the sixth day with sweats. In the phrenitic cases, all the symptoms which have been described did not occur, but in them the disease mostly came to a crisis on the eleventh day, and in some on the twentieth. In those cases in which the phrenitis did not begin immediately, but about the third or fourth day, the disease was moderate at the commencement, but assumed a violent character about the seventh day. There was a great number of diseases, and of those affected, they who died were principally infants, young persons, adults having smooth bodies, white skins, straight and black hair, dark eyes, those living recklessly and luxuriously; persons with shrill, or rough voices, who stammered and were passionate, and women more especially died from this form. In this constitution, four symptoms in particular proved salutary; either a hemorrhage from the nose, or a copious discharge by the bladder of urine, having an abundant and proper sediment, or a bilious disorder of the bowels at the proper time, or an attack of dysentery. And in many cases it happened, that the crisis did not take place by any one of the symptoms which have been mentioned, but the patient passed through most of them, and appeared to be in an uncomfortable way, and yet all who were attacked with these symptoms recovered. All the symptoms which I have described occurred also to women and girls; and whoever of them had any of these symptoms in a favorable manner, or the menses appeared abundantly, were saved thereby, and had a crisis, so that I do not know a single female who had any of these favorably that died. But the daughter of Philo, who had a copious hemorrhage from the nose, and took supper unseasonably on the seventh day, died. In those cases of acute, and more especially of ardent fevers, in which there is an involuntary discharge of tears, you may expect a nasal hemorrhage unless the other symptoms be of a fatal type, for in those of a bad description, they do not indicate a hemorrhage, but death.

12. Swellings about the ears, with pain in fevers, sometimes when the fever went off critically, neither subsided nor were converted into pus; in these cases a bilious diarrhoea, or dysentery, or thick urine having a sediment, carried off the disease, as happened to Hermippus of Clazomenae. The circumstances relating to crises, as far as we can recognize them, were so far similar and so far dissimilar. Thus two brothers became ill at the same hour (they were brothers of Epigenes, and lodged near the theatre), of these the elder had a crisis on the sixth day, and the younger on the seventh, and both had a relapse at the same hour; it then left them for five days, and from the return of the fever both had a crisis together on the seventeenth day. Most had a crisis on the sixth day; it then left them for six days, and from the relapse there was a crisis on the fifth day. But those who had a crisis on the seventh day, had an intermission for seven days; and the crisis took place on the third day after the relapse. Those who had a crisis on the sixth day, after an interval of six days were seized again on the third, and having left them for one day, the fever attacked them again on the next and came to a crisis, as happened to Evagon the son of Daetharses. Those in whom the crisis happened on the sixth day, had an intermission of seven days, and from the relapse there was a crisis on the fourth, as happened to the daughter of Aglaidas. The greater part of those who were taken ill under this constitution of things, were affected in this manner, and I did not know a single case of recovery, in which there was not a relapse agreeably to the stated order of relapses; and all those recovered in which the relapses took place according to this form: nor did I know a single instance of those who then passed through the disease in this manner who had another relapse.

13. In these diseases death generally happened on the sixth day, as with Epaminondas, Silenus, and Philiscus the son of Antagoras. Those who had parotid swellings experienced a crisis on the twentieth day, but in all these cases the disease went off without coming to a suppuration, and was turned upon the bladder. But in Cratistonax, who lived by the temple of Hercules, and in the maid servant of Scymnus the fuller, it turned to a suppuration, and they died. Those who had a crisis on the seventh day, had an intermission of nine days, and a relapse which came to a crisis on the fourth day from the return of the fever, as was

the case with Pantacles, who resided close by the temple of Bacchus. Those who had a crisis on the seventh day, after an interval of six days had a relapse, from which they had a crisis on the seventh day, as happened to Phanocritus, who was lodged with Gnathon the fuller. During the winter, about the winter solstices, and until the equinox, the ardent fevers and frenzies prevailed, and many died. The crisis, however, changed, and happened to the greater number on the fifth day from the commencement, left them for four days and relapsed; and after the return, there was a crisis on the fifth day, making in all fourteen days. The crisis took place thus in the case of most children, also in elder persons. Some had a crisis on the eleventh day, a relapse on the fourteenth, a complete crisis on the twentieth; but certain persons, who had a rigor about the twentieth, had a crisis on the fortieth. The greater part had a rigor along with the original crisis, and these had also a rigor about the crisis in the relapse. There were fewest cases of rigor in the spring, more in summer, still more in autumn, but by far the most in winter; then hemorrhages ceased.

Section Four

1. With regard to diseases, the circumstances from which we form a judgment of them are,- by attending to the general nature of all, and the peculiar nature of each individual,- to the disease, the patient, and the applications,- to the person who applies them, as that makes a difference for better or for worse,- to the whole constitution of the season, and particularly to the state of the heavens, and the nature of each country;- to the patient's habits, regimen, and pursuits;- to his conversation, manners, taciturnity, thoughts, sleep, or absence of sleep, and sometimes his dreams, what and when they occur;- to his picking and scratching;- to his tears;-to the alvine discharges, urine, sputa, and vomitings; and to the changes of diseases from the one into the other;- to the deposits, whether of a deadly or critical character;- to the sweat, coldness, rigor, cough, sneezing, hiccup, respiration, eructation, flatulence, whether passed silently or with a noise;- to hemorrhages and hemorrhoids;- from these, and their consequences, we must form our judgment.

2. Fevers are,- the continual, some of which hold during the day and have a remission at night, and others hold a remission during the day; semi-tertians, tertians, quartans, quintans, septans, nonans. The most

acute, strongest, most dangerous, and fatal diseases, occur in the continual fever. The least dangerous of all, and the mildest and most protracted, is the quartan, for it is not only such from itself, but it also carries off other great diseases. In what is called the semi-tertian, other acute diseases are apt to occur, and it is the most fatal of all others, and moreover phthisical persons, and those laboring under other protracted diseases, are apt to be attacked by it. The nocturnal fever is not very fatal, but protracted; the diurnal is still more protracted, and in some cases passes into phthisis. The septan is protracted, but not fatal; the nonan more protracted, and not fatal. The true tertian comes quickly to a crisis, and is not fatal; but the quintan is the worst of all, for it proves fatal when it precedes an attack of phthisis, and when it supervenes on persons who are already consumptive. There are peculiar modes, and constitutions, and paroxysms, in every one of these fevers; for example,- the continual, in some cases at the very commencement, grows, as it were, and attains its full strength, and rises to its most dangerous pitch, but is diminished about and at the crisis; in others it begins gentle and suppressed, but gains ground and is exacerbated every day, and bursts forth with all its heat about and at the crisis; while in others, again, it commences mildly, increases, and is exacerbated until it reaches its acme, and then remits until at and about the crisis. These varieties occur in every fever, and in every disease. From these observations one must regulate the regimen accordingly. There are many other important symptoms allied to these, part of which have been already noticed, and part will be described afterwards, from a consideration of which one may judge, and decided in each case, whether the disease be acute, acute, and whether it will end in death or recovery; or whether it will be protracted, and will end in death or recovery; and in what cases food is to be given, and in what not; and when and to what amount, and what particular kind of food is to be administered.

3. Those diseases which have their paroxysms on even days have their crises on even days; and those which have their paroxysms on uneven days have their crises on uneven days. The first period of those which have the crisis on even days, is the 4th, 6th, 8th, 10th, 14th, 20th, 30th, 40th, 60th, 80th, 100th; and the first period of those which have their crises on uneven days, is the 1st, 3d, 5th, 7th, 9th, 11th, 17th, 21th, 27th, 31st. It should be known, that if the crisis take place on any other day than on those described, it indicates that there will be a relapse,

which may prove fatal. But one ought to pay attention, and know in these seasons what crises will lead to recovery and what to death, or to changes for the better or the worse. Irregular fevers, quartans, quintans, septans, and nonans should be studied, in order to find out in what periods their crises take place.

Fourteen Cases of Disease

CASE I. Philiscus, who lived by the Wall, took to bed on the first day of acute fever; he sweated; towards night was uneasy. On the second day all the symptoms were exacerbated; late in the evening had a proper stool from a small clyster; the night quiet. On the third day, early in the morning and until noon, he appeared to be free from fever; towards evening, acute fever, with sweating, thirst, tongue parched; passed black urine; night uncomfortable, no sleep; he was delirious on all subjects. On the fourth, all the symptoms exacerbated, urine black; night more comfortable, urine of a better color. On the fifth, about mid-day, had a slight trickling of pure blood from the nose; urine varied in character, having floating in it round bodies, resembling semen, and scattered, but which did not fall to the bottom; a suppository having been applied, some scanty flatulent matters were passed; night uncomfortable, little sleep, talking incoherently; extremities altogether cold, and could not be warmed; urine, black; slept a little towards day; loss of speech, cold sweats; extremities livid; about the middle of the sixth day he died. The respiration throughout, like that of a person recollecting himself, was rare, and large, and spleen was swelled upon in a round tumor, the sweats cold throughout, the paroxysms on the even days.

CASE II. Silenus lived on the Broad-way, near the house of Evalcidas. From fatigue, drinking, and unseasonable exercises, he was seized with fever. He began with having pain in the loins; he had heaviness of the head, and there was stiffness of the neck. On the first day the alvine discharges were bilious, unmixed, frothy, high colored, and copious; urine black, having a black sediment; he was thirsty, tongue dry; no sleep at night. On the second, acute fever, stools more copious, thinner, frothy; urine black, an uncomfortable night, slight delirium. On the third, all the symptoms exacerbated; an oblong distention, of a softish nature, from both sides of the hypochondrium to the navel; stools thin, and darkish; urine muddy, and darkish; no sleep at night;

much talking, laughter, singing, he could not restrain himself. On the fourth, in the same state. On the fifth, stools bilious, unmixed, smooth, greasy; urine thin, and transparent; slight absence of delirium. On the sixth, slight perspiration about the head; extremities cold and livid; much tossing about; no passage from the bowels, urine suppressed, acute fever. On the seventh, loss of speech; extremities could no longer be kept warm; no discharge of urine. On the eighth, a cold sweat all over; red rashes with sweat, of a round figure, small, like vari, persistent, not subsiding; by means of a slight stimulus, a copious discharge from the bowels, of a thin and undigested character, with pain; urine acrid, and passed with pain; extremities slightly heated; sleep slight, and comatose; speechless; urine thin, and transparent. On the ninth, in the same state. On the tenth, no drink taken; comatose, sleep slight; alvine discharges the same; urine abundant, and thickish; when allowed to stand, the sediment farinaceous and white; extremities again cold. On the eleventh, he died. At the commencement, and throughout, the respiration was slow and large; there was a constant throbbing in the hypochondrium; his age was about twenty.

CASE III. Herophon was seized with an acute fever; alvine discharges at first were scanty, and attended with tenesmus; but afterwards they were passed of a thin, bilious character, and frequent; there was no sleep; urine black, and thin. On the fifth, in the morning, deafness; all the symptoms exacerbated; spleen swollen; distention of the hypochondrium; alvine discharges scanty, and black; he became delirious. On the sixth, delirious; at night, sweating, coldness; the delirium continued. On the seventh, he became cold, thirsty, was disordered in mind; at night recovered his senses; slept. On the eighth, was feverish; the spleen diminished in size; quite collected; had pain at first about the groin, on the same side as the spleen; had pains in both legs; night comfortable; urine better colored, had a scanty sediment. On the ninth, sweated; the crisis took place; fever remitted. On the fifth day afterwards, fever relapsed, spleen immediately became swollen; acute fever; deafness again. On the third day after the relapse, the spleen diminished; deafness less; legs painful; sweated during the night; crisis took place on the seventeenth day; had no disorder of the senses during the relapse.

CASE IV. In Thasus, the wife of Philinus, having been delivered of a daughter, the discharge being natural, and other matters going on mildly, on the fourteenth day after delivery was seized with fever, attended with rigor; was pained at first in the cardiac region of the stomach and right hypochondrium; pain in the genital organs; lochial discharge ceased. Upon the application of a pessary all these symptoms were alleviated; pains of the head, neck, and loins remained; no sleep; extremities cold; thirst; bowels in a hot state; stools scanty; urine thin, and colorless at first. On the sixth, towards night, senses much disordered, but again were restored. On the seventh, thirsty; the evacuations bilious, and high colored. On the eighth, had a rigor; acute fever; much spasm, with pain; talked much, incoherently; upon the application of a suppository, rose to stool, and passed copious dejections, with a bilious flux; no sleep. On the ninth, spasms. On the tenth, slightly recollected. On the eleventh, slept; had perfect recollection, but again immediately wandered; passed a large quantity of urine with spasms, (the attendants seldom putting her in mind), it was thick, white, like urine which has been shaken after it has stood for a considerable time until it has subsided, but it had no sediment; in color and consistence, the urine resembled that of cattle, as far as I observed. About the fourteenth day, startings over the whole body; talked much; slightly collected, but presently became again delirious. About the seventeenth day became speechless, on the twentieth died.

CASE V. The wife of Epicrates, who was lodged at the house of Archigetes, being near the term of delivery, was seized with a violent rigor, and, as was said, she did not become heated; next day the same. On the third, she was delivered of a daughter, and everything went on properly. On the day following her delivery, she was seized with acute fever, pain in the cardiac region of the stomach, and in the genital parts. Having had a suppository, was in so far relieved; pain in the head, neck, and loins; no sleep; alvine discharges scanty, bilious, thin, and unmixed; urine thin, and blackish. Towards the night of the sixth day from the time she was seized with the fever, became delirious. On the seventh, all the symptoms exacerbated; insomnolency, delirium, thirst; stools bilious, and high colored. On the eighth, had a rigor; slept more. On the ninth, the same. On the tenth, her limbs painfully affected; pain again of the cardiac region of the stomach; heaviness of the head; no delirium; slept more; bowels constipated. On the eleventh, passed urine of a better color, and having an abundant sediment; felt lighter. On the fourteenth had a rigor; acute fever. On the fifteenth, had a copious vomiting of bilious and yellow matters; sweated; fever gone; at night acute fever; urine thick, sediment white. On the seventeenth, an exacerbation; night uncomfortable; no sleep; delirium. On the eighteenth, thirsty; tongue parched; no sleep; much delirium; legs painfully affected. About the twentieth, in the morning, had as light rigor; was comatose; slept tranquilly; had slight vomiting of bilious and black matters; towards night deafness. About the twenty-first, weight generally in the left side, with pain; slight urine thick, muddy, and reddish; when allowed to stand, had no sediment; in other respects felt lighter; fever not gone; fauces painful from the commencement, and red; uvula retracted; defluxion remained acrid, pungent, and saltish throughout. About the twenty-seventh, free of fever; sediment in the urine; pain in the side. About the thirty-first, was attacked with fever, bilious diarrhea; slight bilious vomiting on the fortieth. Had a complete crisis, and was freed from the fever on the eightieth day.

CASE VI. Cleonactides, who was lodged above the Temple of Hercules, was seized with a fever in an irregular form; was pained in the head and left side from the commencement, and had other pains resembling those produced by fatigue; paroxysms of the fevers inconstant and irregular; occasional sweats; the paroxysms generally attacked on the critical days. About the twenty-fourth was cold in the extremities of the hands, vomitings bilious, yellow, and frequent, soon turning to a verdigris-green color; general relief. About the thirtieth, began to have hemorrhage from both nostrils, and this continued in an irregular manner until near the crisis; did not loathe food, and had no thirst throughout, nor was troubled with insomnolency; urine thin, and not devoid of color. When about the thirtieth day, passed reddish urine, having a copious red sediment; was relieved, but afterwards the characters of the urine varied, sometimes having sediment, and sometimes not. On the sixtieth, the sediment in the urine copious, white, and smooth; all the symptoms ameliorated; intermission of the fever; urine thin, and well colored. On the seventieth, fever gone for ten days. On the eightieth had a rigor, was seized with acute fever, sweated much; a red, smooth sediment in the urine; and a perfect crisis.

CASE VII. Meton was seized with fever; there was a painful weight in the loins. Next day, after drinking water pretty copiously, had proper evacuations from the bowels. On the third, heaviness of the head, stools thin, bilious, and reddish. On the fourth, all the symptoms exacerbated; had twice a scanty trickling of blood from the right nostril;

passed an uncomfortable night; alvine discharges like those on the third day; urine darkish, had a darkish cloud floating in it, of a scattered form, which did not subside. On the fifth, a copious hemorrhage of pure blood from the left he sweated, and had a crisis. After the fever restless, and had some delirium; urine thin, and darkish; had an affusion of warm water on the head; slept and recovered his senses. In this case there was no relapse, but there were frequent hemorrhages after the crisis.

CASE VIII. Erasinus, who lived near the Canal of Bootes, was seized with fever after supper; passed the night in an agitated state. During the first day quiet, but in pain at night. On the second, symptoms all exacerbated; at night delirious. On the third, was in a painful condition; great incoherence. On the fourth, in a most uncomfortable state; had no sound sleep at night, but dreaming and talking; then all the appearances worse, of a formidable and alarming character; fear, impatience. On the morning of the fifth, was composed, and quite coherent, but long before noon was furiously mad, so that he could not constrain himself; extremities cold, and somewhat livid; urine without sediment; died about sunset. The fever in this case was accompanied by sweats throughout; the sweats throughout; the hypochondria were in a state of meteorism, with distention and pain; the urine was black, has round substances floating in it, which did not subside; the alvine evacuations were not stopped; thirst throughout not great; much spasms with sweats about the time of death.

CASE IX. Criton, in Thasus, while still on foot, and going about, was seized with a violent pain in the great toe; he took to bed the same day, had rigors and nausea, recovered his heat slightly, at night was delirious. On the second, swelling of the whole foot, and about the ankle erythema, with distention, and small bullae (phlyctaenae); acute fever; he became furiously deranged; alvine discharges bilious, unmixed, and rather frequent. He died on the second day from the commencement.

CASE X. The Clazomenian who was lodged by the Well of Phrynichides was seized with fever. He had pain in the head, neck, and loins from the beginning, and immediately afterwards deafness; no sleep, acute fever, hypochondria elevated with a swelling, but not much distention; tongue dry. On the fourth, towards night, he became delirious. On the fifth, in an uneasy state. On the sixth, all the symptoms exacerbated. About the eleventh a slight remission; from the commencement to the fourteenth day the alvine discharges thin, copious, and of the color of water, but were well supported; the bowels then became constipated. Urine throughout thin, and well colored, and had many substances scattered through it, but no sediment. About the sixteenth, urine somewhat thicker, which had a slight sediment; somewhat better, and more collected. On the seventeenth, urine again thin; swellings about both his ears, with pain; no sleep, some incoherence; legs painfully affected. On the twentieth, free of fever, had a crisis, no sweat, perfectly collected. About the twenty-seventh, violent pain of the right hip; it speedily went off. The swellings about the ears subsided, and did not suppurate, but were painful. About the thirty-first, a diarrhea attended with a copious discharge of watery matter, and symptoms of dysentery; passed thick urine; swellings about the ears gone. About the fortieth day, had pain in the right eye, sight dull. It went away.

CASE XI. The wife of Dromeades having been delivered of a female child, and all other matters going on properly, on the second day after was seized with rigor and acute fever. Began to have pain about the hypochondrium on the first day; had nausea and incoherence, and for some hours afterwards had no sleep; respiration rare, large, and suddenly interrupted. On the day following that on which she had the rigor, alvine discharges proper; urine thick, white, muddy, like urine which has been shaken after standing for some time, until the sediment had fallen to the bottom; it had no sediment; she did not sleep during the night. On the third day, about noon, had a rigor, acute fever; urine the same; pain of the hypochondria, nausea, an uncomfortable night, no sleep; a coldish sweat all over, but heat quickly restored. On the fourth, slight alleviation of the symptoms about the hypochondria; heaviness of the head, with pain; somewhat comatose; slight epistaxis, tongue dry, thirst, urine thin and oily; slept a little, upon awaking was somewhat comatose; slight coldness, slept during the night, was delirious. On the morning of the sixth had a rigor, but soon recovered her heat, sweated all over; extremities cold, was delirious, respiration rare and large. Shortly afterwards spasms from the head began, and she immediately expired.

CASE XII. A man, in a heated state, took supper, and drank more than enough; he vomited the whole during the night; acute fever, pain of the right hypochondrium, a softish inflammation from the inner part; passed an uncomfortable night; urine at the commencement thick, red, but when allowed to stand, had no sediment, tongue dry, and not very thirsty. On the fourth, acute fever, pains all over. On the fifth, urine smooth, oily, and copious; acute fever. On the sixth, in the evening, very incoherent, no sleep during the night. On the seventh, all the symptoms exacerbated; urine of the same characters; much talking, and he could not contain himself; the bowels being stimulated, passed a watery discharge with lumbrici: night equally painful. In the morning had a rigor; acute fever, hot sweat, appeared to be free of fever; did not sleep long; after the sleep a chill, ptyalism; in the evening, great incoherence; after a little, vomited a small quantity of dark bilious matters. On the ninth, coldness, much delirium, did not sleep. On the tenth, pains in the limbs, all the symptoms exacerbated; he was delirious. On the eleventh, he died.

CASE XIII. A woman, who lodged on the Quay, being three months gone with child, was seized with fever, and immediately began to have pains in the loins. On the third day, pain of the head and neck, extending to the clavicle, and right hand; she immediately lost the power of speech; was paralyzed in the right hand, with spasms, after the manner of paraplegia; was quite incoherent; passed an uncomfortable night; did not sleep; disorder of the bowels, attended with bilious, On the fourth, recovered the use of her tongue; spasms of the same parts, and general pains remained; swelling in the hypochondrium, accompanied with pain; did not sleep, was quite incoherent; bowels disordered, urine thin, and not of a good color. On the fifth, acute fever; pain of the hypochondrium, quite incoherent; alvine evacuations bilious; towards night had a sweat, and was freed from the fever. On the sixth, recovered her reason; was every way relieved; the pain remained about the left clavicle; was thirsty, urine thin, had no sleep. On the seventh trembling, slight coma, some incoherence, pains about the clavicle and left arm remained; in all other respects was alleviated; quite coherent. For three days remained free from fever. On the eleventh, had a relapse, with rigor and fever. About the fourteenth day, vomited pretty abundantly bilious and yellow matters, had a sweat, the fever went off, by coming to a crisis.

CASE XIV. Melidia, who lodged near the Temple of Juno, began to feel a violent pain of the head, neck, and chest. She was straightway seized with acute fever; a slight appearance of the menses; continued pains of all these parts. On the sixth, was affected with coma, nausea, and rigor; redness about the cheeks; slight delirium. On the seventh, had a sweat; the fever intermitted, the pains remained. A relapse; little sleep; urine throughout of a good color, but thin; the alvine evacuations were thin, bilious, acrid, very scanty, black, and fetid; a white, smooth sediment in the urine; had a sweat, and experienced a perfect crisis on the eleventh day.

Book II

Section One

CASE I. Pythion, who lived by the Temple of the Earth, on the first day, trembling commencing from his hands; acute fever, delirium. On the second, all the symptoms were exacerbated. On the third, the same. On the fourth alvine discharges scanty, unmixed, and bilious. On the fifth, all the symptoms were exacerbated, the tremors remained; little sleep, the bowels constipated. On the sixth sputa mixed, reddish. On the seventh, mouth drawn aside. On the eighth, all the symptoms were exacerbated; the tremblings were again constant; urine, from the beginning to the eighth day, thin, and devoid of color; substances floating in it, cloudy. On the tenth he sweated; sputa somewhat digested, had a crisis; urine thinnish about the crisis; but after the crisis, on the fortieth day, an abscess about the anus, which passed off by a strangury.

Explanation of the characters. It is probably that the great discharge of urine brought about the resolution of the disease, and the cure of the patient on the fortieth day. CASE II. Hermocrates, who lived by the New Wall, was seized with fever. He began to have pain in the head and loins; an empty distention of the hypochondrium; the tongue at first was parched; deafness at the commencement; there was no sleep; not very thirsty; urine thick and red, when allowed to stand it did not subside; alvine discharge very dry, and not scanty. On the fifth, urine thin, had substances floating in it which did not fall to the bottom; at night he was delirious. On the sixth, had jaundice; all the symptoms were exacerbated; had no recollection. On the seventh, in an uncomfortable state; urine thin, as formerly; on the following days the same. About the eleventh day, all the symptoms appeared to be lightened. Coma set in; urine thicker, reddish, thin substances below, had no sediment; by degrees he became collected. On the fourteenth, fever gone; had no sweat; slept, quite collected; urine of the same characters. About the seventeenth, had a relapse, became hot. On the following days, acute fever, urine thin, was delirious. Again, on the twentieth, had a crisis; free of fever; had no sweat; no appetite through the whole time; was perfectly collected; could not speak, tongue dry, without thirst; deep sleep. About the twenty-fourth day he became heated; bowels loose, with a thin, watery discharge; on the following days acute fever, tongue parched. On the twenty-seventh he died. In this patient deafness continued throughout; the urine either thick and red, without sediment, or thin, devoid of color, and, having substances floating in it: he could taste nothing. Explanation of the characters. It is probably that it was the suppression of the discharges from the bowels which occasioned death on the twenty-seventh day.

CASE III. The man who was lodged in the Garden of Dealces: had heaviness of the head and pain in the right temple for a considerable time, from some accidental cause, was seized with fever, and took to bed. On the second, there was a trickling of pure blood from the left nostril, but the alvine discharges were proper, urine thin, mixed, having small substances floating in it, like coarse barley meal, or semen. On the third, acute fever; stools black, thin, frothy, a livid sediment in the dejections; slight coma; uneasiness at the times he had to get up; sediment in the urine livid, and somewhat viscid. On the fourth, slight vomiting of bilious, yellow matters, and, after a short interval, of the color of verdigris; a few drops of pure blood ran from the left nostril; stools the same; urine the same; sweated about the head and clavicles; spleen enlarged, pain of the thigh on the same side; loose swelling of the right hypochondrium; at night had no sleep, slight delirium. On the sixth, stools black, fatty, viscid, fetid; slept, more collected. On the seventh, tongue dry, thirsty, did not sleep; was somewhat delirious; urine thin, not of a good color. On the eighth, stools black, scanty, and compact; slept, became collected; not very thirsty. On the ninth had a rigor, acute fever, sweated, a chill, was delirious, strabismus of the right eye, tongue dry, thirsty, without sleep. On the tenth, much the same. On the eleventh, became quite collected; free from fever, slept, urine thin about the crisis. The two following days without fever; it returned on the fourteenth, then immediately insomnolency and complete delirium. On the fifteenth, urine muddy, like that which has been shaken after the sediment has fallen to the bottom; acute fever, quite delirious, did not sleep; knees and legs painful; after a suppository, had alvine dejections of a black color. On the sixteenth, urine thin, had a cloudy eneorema, was delirious. On the seventeenth, in the morning, extremities cold, was covered up with the bedclothes, acute fever, general sweat, felt relieved, more collected; not free of fever, thirsty, vomited yellow bile, in small quantities; formed faeces passed from the bowels, but soon afterwards black, scanty, and thin; urine thin, not well colored. On the eighteenth, not collected, comatose. On the nineteenth, in the same state. On the twentieth, slept; quite collected, sweated, free from fever, not thirsty, but the urine thin. On the twenty-first, slight delirium; somewhat thirsty, pain of the hypochondrium, and throbbing about the navel throughout. On sediment in the urine, quite collected. Twenty-seventh, pain of the right hip joint; urine thin and bad, a sediment; all the other symptoms milder. About the twenty-ninth, pain of the right eye; urine thin. Fortieth, dejections pituitous, white, rather frequent; sweated abundantly all over; had a complete crisis.

Explanation of the characters. It is probable that, by means of the stools, the urine, and the sweat, this patient was cured in forty days.

Section Two

CASE I. In Thasus, Philistes had headache of long continuance, and sometimes was confined to bed, with a tendency to deep sleep; having been seized with continual fevers from drinking, the pain was exacerbated; during the night he, at first, became hot. On the first day, he vomited some bilious matters, at first yellow, but afterwards of a verdigris-green color, and in greater quantity; formed faeces passed from the bowels; passed the night uncomfortably. On the second, deafness, acute fever; retraction of the right hypochondrium; urine thin, transparent, had some small substances like semen floating in it; delirium ferox about mid-day. On the third, in an uncomfortable state. On the fourth, convulsions; all the symptoms exacerbated. On the fifth, early in the morning, died. Explanation of the characters. It is probable that the death of the patient on the fifth day is to be attributed to a phrenitis, with unfavorable evacuations.

CASE II. Charion, who was lodged at the house of Demaenetus, contracted a fever from drinking. Immediately he had a painful heaviness of the head; did not sleep; bowels disordered, with thin and somewhat bilious discharges. On the third day, acute fever; trembling of the head, but especially of the lower lip; after a little time a rigor, convulsions; he was quite delirious; passed the night uncomfortably. On the fourth, quiet, slept little, talked incoherently. On the fifth, in pain; all the symptoms exacerbated; delirium; passed the night uncomfortably; did not sleep. On the sixth, in the same state. On the seventh had a rigor, acute fever, sweated all over his body; had a crisis. Throughout the alvine discharges were bilious, scanty, and unmixed; urine thin, well colored, having cloudy substances floating in it. About the eighth day, passed urine of a better color, having a white scanty sediment; was collected, free from fever for a season. On the ninth it relapsed. About the fourteenth, acute fever. On the sixteenth, vomited pretty frequently yellow, bilious matters. On the seventeenth had a rigor, acute fever, sweated, free of fever; had a crisis; urine, after the relapse and the crisis, well colored, having a sediment; neither was he delirious in the relapse. On the eighteenth, became a little heated; some thirst, urine thin, with cloudy substances floating in it; slight wandering in his mind. About the nineteenth, free of fever, had a pain in his neck; a sediment in the urine. Had a complete crisis on the twentieth. Explanation of the characters. It is probable that the patient was cured in twenty days, by the abundance of bilious stools and urine.

CASE III. The daughter of Euryanax, a maid, was taken ill of fever. She was free of thirst throughout, but had no relish for food. Alvine discharges small, urine thin, scanty, not well colored. In the beginning of the fever, had a pain about the nates. On the sixth day, was free of fever, did not sweat, had a crisis; the complaint about the nates came to a small suppuration, and burst at the crisis. After the crisis, on the seventh day, had a rigor, became slightly heated, sweated. On the eighth day after the rigor, had an inconsiderable rigor; the extremities cold ever after. About the tenth day, after a sweat which came on, she became delirious, and again immediately afterwards was collected; these symptoms were said to have been brought on by eating grapes. After an intermission of the twelfth day, she again talked much incoherently; her bowels disordered with bilious, scanty, unmixed, thin, acrid discharges; she required to get frequently up. She died on the seventh day after the return of the delirium. At the commencement of the disease she had pain in the throat, and it red throughout, uvula retracted, defluxions abundant, thin, acrid; coughed, but had no concocted sputa; during the whole time loathed all kinds of food, nor had the least desire of anything; had no thirst, nor drank anything worth mentioning; was silent, and never spoke a word; despondency; had no hopes of herself. She had a congenital tendency to phthisis.

CASE IV. The woman affected with quinsy, who lodged in the house of Aristion: her complaint began in the tongue; speech inarticulate; tongue red and parched. On the first day, felt chilly, and afterwards became heated. On the third day, a rigor, acute fever; a reddish and hard swelling on both sides of the neck and chest, extremities cold and livid; and livid; respiration elevated; the drink returned by the nose; she could not swallow; alvine and urinary discharges suppressed. On the fourth, all of the symptoms were exacerbated. On the fifth she died of the quinsy. Explanation of the characters. It is probable that the cause of death on the sixth day was the suppression of the discharges.

CASE V. The young man who was lodged by the Liars' Market was seized with fever from fatigue, labor, and running out of season. On the first day, the bowels disordered, with bilious, thin, and copious dejections; urine thin and blackish; had no sleep; was thirsty. On the second all the symptoms were exacerbated; dejections more copious and unseasonable; he had no sleep; disorder of the intellect; slight sweat. On the third day, restless, thirst, nausea, much tossing about, bewilderment, delirium; extremities livid and cold; softish distention of the hypochondrium on both sides. On the fourth, did not sleep; still worse. On the seventh he died. He was about twenty years of age. Explanation of the characters. It is probable that the cause of his death on the seventh day was the unseasonable practices mentioned above. An acute affection.

CASE VI. The woman who lodged at the house of Tisamenas had a troublesome attack of iliac passion, much vomiting; could not keep her drink; pains about the hypochondria, and pains also in the lower part of the belly; constant tormina; not thirsty; became hot; extremities cold throughout, with nausea and insomnolency; urine scanty and thin; dejections undigested, thin, scanty. Nothing could do her any good. She died.

CASE VII. A woman of Pantimides, from a miscarriage, was taken ill of fever. On the first day, tongue dry, thirst, nausea, insomnolency, belly disordered, with thin, copious, undigested dejections. On the second day, had a rigor, acute fever; alvine discharges copious; had no sleep. On the third, pains greater. On the fourth, delirious. On the seventh she died. Belly throughout loose, with copious, thin, undigested evacuations; urine scanty, thin. An ardent fever.

CASE VIII. Another woman, after a miscarriage about the fifth month, the wife of Ocetes, was seized with fever. At first had sometimes coma and sometimes insomnolency; pain of the loins; heaviness of the head. On the second, the bowels were disordered, with scanty, thin, and at first unmixed dejections. On the third, more copious, and worse; at night did not sleep. On the fourth was delirious; frights, despondency; strabismus of the right eye; a faint cold sweat about the head; extremities cold. On the fifth day, all the symptoms were exacerbated; talked much incoherently, and again immediately became collected; had no thirst; labored under insomnolency; alvine dejections copious, and unseasonable throughout; urine scanty, thin, darkish; extremities cold, somewhat livid. On the sixth day, in the same state. On the seventh she died. Phrenitis.

CASE IX. A woman who lodged near the Liars' Market, having then brought forth a son in a first and difficult labor, was seized with fever. Immediately on the commencement had thirst, nausea, and cardialgia; tongue dry; bowels disordered, with thin and scanty dejections; had no sleep. On the second, had slight rigor, acute fever; a faint cold sweat about the head. On the third, painfully affected; evacuations from the bowels undigested, thin, and copious. On the fourth, had a rigor; all the symptoms exacerbated; insomnolency. On the fifth, in a painful state. On the sixth, in the same state; discharges from the bowels liquid and copious. On the seventh, had a rigor, fever acute; much thirst; much tossing about; towards evening a cold sweat over all; extremities cold, could no longer be kept warm; and again at night had a rigor; extremities could not be warmed; she did not sleep; was slightly delirious, and again speedily collected. On the eighth, about mid-day, she became warm, was thirsty, comatose, had nausea; vomited small quantities of yellowish bile; restless at night, did not sleep; passed frequently large quantities of urine without consciousness. On the ninth, all the symptoms gave way; comatose, towards evening slight rigors; small vomitings of bile. On the tenth, rigor; exacerbation of the fever, did not sleep at all; in the morning passed much urine having a sediment; extremities recovered their heat. On the eleventh, vomited bile of a verdigris-green color; not long after had a rigor, and again the extremities cold; towards evening a rigor, a cold sweat, much vomiting; passed a painful night. On the twelfth, had copious black and fetid vomitings; much hiccup, painful thirst. On the thirteenth, vomitings black, fetid, and copious; rigor about mid-day, loss of speech. On the fourteenth, some blood ran from her nose, she died. In this case the bowels were loose throughout; with rigors: her age about seventeen. An ardent fever.

Section Three

1. The year was southerly, rainy; no winds throughout. Droughts having prevailed during the previous seasons of the year, the south winds towards the rising of Arcturus were attended with much rain. Autumn gloomy and cloudy, with copious rains. Winter southerly, damp, and soft. But long after the solstice, and near the equinox, much wintery weather out of season; and when now close to the equinox, northerly, and winterly weather for no long time. The spring again southerly, calm, much rain until the dog-days. Summer fine and hot; great suffocating heats. The Etesian winds blew small and irregular; again, about the season of Arcturus, much rains with north winds.

2. The year being southerly, damp, and soft towards winter, all were healthy, except those affected with phthisis, of whom we shall write afterwards. 3. Early in spring, along with the prevailing cold, there were many cases of erysipelas, some from a manifest cause, and some not. They were of a malignant nature, and proved fatal to many; many had sore-throat and loss of speech. There were many cases of ardent fever, phrensy, aphthous affections of the mouth, tumors on the genital organs; of ophthalmia, anthrax, disorder of the bowels, anorexia, with thirst and without it; of disordered urine, large in quantity, and bad in quality; of persons affected with coma for a long time, and then falling into a state of insomnolency. There were many cases of failure of crisis, and many of unfavorable crisis; many of dropsy and of phthisis. Such were the diseases then epidemic. There were patients affected with every one of the species which have been mentioned, and many died. The symptoms in each of these cases were as follows:

4. In many cases erysipelas, from some obvious cause, such as an accident, and sometimes from even a very small wound, broke out all over the body, especially, in persons about sixty years of age, about the head, if such an accident was neglected in the slightest degree; and this happened in some who were under treatment; great inflammation took place, and the erysipelas quickly spread all over. in the most of them abscessed ended in suppurations, and there were great fallings off (sloughing) of the flesh, tendons, and bones; and the defluxion which seated in the part was not like pus, but a sort of putrefaction, and the running was large and of various characters. Those cases in which any of these things happened about the head were accompanied with falling off of the hairs of the head and chin, the bones were laid bare and separated, and there were excessive runnings; and these symptoms happened in fevers and without fevers. But these things were more formidable in appearance than dangerous; for when the concoction in these cases turned to a these cases turned to a suppuration, most of them recovered; but when the inflammation and erysipelas disappeared, and when no abscess was formed, a great number of these died. In like manner, the same things happened to whatever part of the body the disease wandered, for in many cases both forearm and arm dropped off; and in those cases in which it fell upon the sides, the parts there, either before or behind, got into a bad state; and in some cases the whole femur and bones of the leg and whole foot were laid bare. But of all such cases, the most formidable were those which took place about the pubes and genital organs. Such was the nature of these cases when attended with sores, and proceeding from an external cause; but the same things occurred in fevers, before fevers, and after fevers. fevers. But those cases in which an abscess was formed, and turned to a suppuration, or a seasonable diarrhea or discharge of good urine took place, were relieved thereby: but those cases in which none of these symptoms occurred, but they disappeared without a crisis, proved fatal. The greater number of these erysipelatous cases took place in the spring, but were prolonged through the summer and during autumn.

5. In certain cases there was much disorder, and tumors about the fauces, and inflammations of the tongue, and abscesses about the teeth. And many were attacked with impairment or loss of speech; at first, those in the commencement of phthisis, but also persons in ardent fever and in phrenitis.

6. The cases of ardent fever and phrenitis occurred early in spring after the cold set in, and great numbers were taken ill at that time, and these cases were attended with acute and fatal symptoms. The constitution of the ardent fevers which then occurred was as follows: at the commencement they were affected with coma, nausea, and rigors; fever acute, not much thirst, nor delirium, slight epistaxis, the paroxysms for the most part on even days; and, about the time of the paroxysms, forgetfulness, loss of strength and of speech, the extremities, that is to say, the hands and feet, at all times, but more especially about the time of the paroxysms, were colder than natural; they slowly and imperfectly became warmed, and again recovered their recollection and speech. They were constantly affected either with coma, in which they got which they got no sleep, or with insomnolency, attended with pains; most had disorders of the bowels, attended with undigested, thin, and copious evacuations; urine copious, thin, having nothing critical nor favorable about it; neither was there any other critical appearance in persons affected thus; for neither was there any proper hemorrhage, nor any other of the accustomed evacuations, to prove a crisis. They died, as it happened, in an irregular manner, mostly about the crisis, but in some instances after having lost their speech for a long time, and having had copious sweats. These were the symptoms which marked the fatal cases of ardent fever; similar symptoms occurred in the phrenitic cases; but these were particularly free from thirst, and none of these had wild delirium as in other cases, but they died oppressed by a bad tendency to sleep, and stupor.

7. But there were also other fevers, as will be described. Many had their mouths affected with aphthous ulcerations. There were also many defluxions about the genital parts, and ulcerations, boils (phymata), externally and internally, about the groins. Watery ophthalmies of a chronic character, with pains; fungous excrescences of the eyelids, externally and internally, called fig, which destroyed the sight of many persons. There were fungous growths, in many other instances, on ulcers, especially on those seated on the genital organs. There were many attacks of carbuncle (anthrax) through the summer, and other affections, which are called "the putrefaction" (seps); also large ecthymata, and large tetters (herpetes) in many instances.

8. And many and serious complaints attacked many persons in the region of the belly. In the first place, tenesmus, accompanied with pain,

attacked many, but more especially children, and all who had not attained to puberty; and the most of these died. There were many cases of lientery and of dysentery; but these were not attended with much pain. The evacuations were bilious, and fatty, and thin, and watery; in many instances the disease terminated in this way, with and without fever; there were painful tormina and volvuli of a malignant kind; copious evacuations of the contents of the guts, and yet much remained behind; and the passages did not carry off the pains, but yielded with difficulty to the means administered; for in most cases purgings were hurtful to those affected in this manner; many died speedily, but in many others they held out longer. In a word, all died, both those who had acute attacks and those who had chronic, most especially from affections of the belly, for it was the belly which carried them all off.

9. All persons had an aversion to food in all the afore-mentioned complaints to a degree such as I never met with before, and persons in these complaints most especially, and those recovering from them, and in all other diseases of a mortal nature. Some were troubled with thirst, and some not; and both in febrile complaints and in others no one drank unseasonably or disobeyed injunctions.

10. The urine in many cases was not in proportion to the drink administered, but greatly in excess; and the badness of the urine voided was great, for it had not the proper thickness, nor concoction, nor purged properly; for in many cases purgings by the bladder indicate favorably, but in the greatest number they indicated a melting of the body, disorder of the bowels, pains, and a want of crisis.

11. Persons laboring under phrenitis and causus were particularly disposed to coma; but also in all other great diseases which occurred along with fever. In the main, most cases were attended either by heavy coma, or by short and light sleep.

12. And many other forms of fevers were then epidemic, of tertian, of quartan, of nocturnal, of continual, of chronic, of erratic, of fevers attended with nausea, and of irregular fevers. All these were attended with much disorder, for the bowels in most cases were disordered, accompanied with rigors, sweats not of a critical character, and with the state of the urine as described. In most instances the disease was protracted, for neither did the deposits which took place prove critical

as in other cases; for in all complaints and in all cases there was difficulty of crisis, want of crisis, and protraction of the disease, but most especially in these. A few had the crisis about the eightieth day, but in most instances it (the disease?) left them irregularly. A few of them died of dropsy without being confined to bed. And in many other diseases people were troubled with swelling, but more especially in phthisical cases.

13. The greatest and most dangerous disease, and the one that proved fatal to the greatest number, was consumption. With many persons it commenced during the winter, and of these some were confined to bed, and others bore up on foot; the most of those died early in spring who were confined to bed; of the others, the cough left not a single person, but it became milder through the summer; during the autumn, all these were confined to bed, and many of them died, but in the greater number of cases the disease was long protracted. Most of these were suddenly attacked with these diseases, having frequent rigors, often continual and acute fevers; unseasonable, copious, and cold sweats throughout; great coldness, from which they had great difficulty in being restored to heat; the bowels variously constipated, and again immediately in a loose state, but towards the termination in all cases with violent looseness of the bowels; a determination downwards of all matters collected about the lungs; urine excessive, and not good; troublesome melting. The coughs throughout were frequent, and copious, digested, and liquid, but not brought up with much pain; and even when they had some slight pain, in all cases the purging of the matters about the lungs went on mildly. The fauces were not very irritable, nor were they troubled with any saltish humors; but there were viscid, white, liquid, frothy, and copious defluxions from the head. But by far the greatest mischief attending these and the other complaints, was the aversion to food, as has been described. For neither been described. For neither had they any relish for drink along with their food, but continued without thirst. There was heaviness of the body, disposition to coma, in most cases swelling, which ended in dropsy; they had rigors, and were delirious towards death.

14. The form of body peculiarly subject to phthisical complaints was the smooth, the whitish, that resembling the lentil; the reddish, the blue-eyed, the leucophlegmatic, and that with the scapulae having the appearance of wings: and women in like manner, with regard to the

melancholic and subsanguineous, phrenitic and dysenteric affections principally attacked them. Tenesmus troubled young persons of a phlegmatic temperament. Chronic diarrhoea, acrid and viscid discharges from the bowels, attacked those who were troubled with bitter bile.

15. To all those which have been described, the season of spring was most inimical, and proved fatal to the greatest numbers: the summer was the most favorable to them, and the fewest died then; in autumn, and under the Pleiades, again there died great numbers. It appears to me, according to the reason of things, that the coming on of summer should have done good in these cases; for winter coming on cures the diseases of summer, and summer coming on removes the diseases of winter. And yet the summer in question was not of itself well constituted, for it became suddenly hot, southerly, and calm; but, not withstanding, it proved beneficial by producing a change on the other constitution.

16. I look upon it as being a great part of the art to be able to judge properly of that which has been written. For he that knows and makes a proper use of these things, would appear to me not likely to commit any great mistake in the art. He ought to learn accurately the constitution of every one of the seasons, and of the diseases; whatever that is common in each constitution and disease is good, and whatever is bad; whatever disease will be protracted and end in death, and whatever will be protracted and end in recovery; which disease of an acute nature will end in death, and which in recovery. From these it is easy to know the order of the critical days, and prognosticate from them accordingly. And to a person who is skilled in these things, it is easy to know to whom, when, and how aliment ought to be administered.

Sixteen Cases of Disease

CASE I. In Thasus, the Parian who lodged above the Temple of Diana was seized with an acute fever, at first of a continual and ardent type; thirsty, inclined to be comatose at first, and afterwards troubled with insomnolency; bowels disordered at the beginning, urine thin. On the sixth day, passed oily urine, was delirious. On the seventh, all the symptoms were exacerbated; had no sleep, but the urine of the same characters, and the understanding disordered; alvine dejections bilious and fatty. On the eighth, a slight epistaxis; small vomiting of verdigris-green matters; slept a little. On the ninth, in the same state. On the tenth, all the symptoms gave way. On the eleventh, he sweated, but not over the whole body; he became cold, but immediately recovered his heat again. On the fourteenth, acute fever; discharges bilious, thin, and copious; substances floating in the urine; he became incoherent. On the seventeenth, in a painful state, for he had no sleep, and the fever was more intense. On the twentieth, sweated all over; apyrexia, dejections bilious; aversion to food, comatose. On the twenty-fourth, had a relapse. On the thirty-fourth, apyrexia; bowels not confined; and he again recovered his heat. Fortieth, apyrexia, bowels confined for no long time, aversion to food; had again slight symptoms of fever, and throughout in an irregular form; apyrexia at times, and at others not; for if the fever intermitted, and was alleviated for a little, it immediately relapsed again; he used much and improper food; sleep bad; about the time of the relapse he was delirious; passed thick urine at that time, but troubled, and of bad characters; bowels at first confined, and again loose; slight fevers of a continual type; discharges copious and thin. On the hundred and twentieth day he died. In this patient the bowels were constantly from the first either loose, with bilious, liquid, and copious dejections, or constipated with hot and undigested faeces; the urine throughout bad; for the most part coma, or insomnolency with pain; continued aversion to food. Ardent fever. Explanation of the characters. It is probable that the weakness produced by the fever, the phrenitis, and affection of the hypochondrium caused death on the hundred and twentieth day.

CASE II. In Thasus, the woman who lodged near the Cold Water, on the third day after delivery of a daughter, the lochial discharge not taking place, was seized with acute fever, accompanied with rigors. But a considerable time before delivery she was feverish, confined to bed, and loathed her food. After the rigor which took place, continual and acute fevers, with rigors. On the eighth and following days, was very incoherent, and immediately afterwards became collected; bowels disordered, with copious, thin, watery, and bilious stools; no thirst. On the eleventh was collected, but disposed to coma; urine copious, thin, and black; no sleep. On the twentieth, slight chills, and immediately afterwards was warm; slight incoherence; no sleep; with regard to the bowels, in the same condition; urine watery, and copious. On the twenty-seventh, free from fever; bowels constipated; not long afterwards violent pain of the right hip-joint for a considerable time; fevers afterwards supervened; urine watery. On the fortieth, complaints about the hip-joint better; continued coughs, with copious, watery sputa; bowels constipated; aversion to food; urine the same; fever not leaving her entirely, but having paroxysms in an irregular form, sometimes present, sometimes not. On the sixtieth, the coughs left her without a crisis, for no concoction of the sputa took place, nor any of the usual abscesses; jaw on the right side convulsively retracted; comatose, was again incoherent, and immediately became collected; utter aversion to food; the jaw became relaxed; alvine discharges small, and bilious; fever more acute, affected with rigors; on the following days lost her speech, and again became collected, and talked. On the eightieth she died. In this case the urine throughout was black, thin, and watery; coma supervened; there was aversion to food, aversion to food, despondency, and insomnolency; irritability, restlessness; she was of a melancholic turn of mind. Explanation of the characters. It is probable that the suppression of the lochial discharge caused death on the day.

CASE III. In Thasus, Pythion, who was lodged above the Temple of Hercules, from labor, fatigue, and neglected diet, was seized with strong rigor and acute fever; tongue dry, thirsty, and bilious; had no sleep; urine darkish, eneorema floating on the top of the urine, did not subside. On the second day, about noon, coldness of the extremities, especially about the hands and head; loss of speech and of articulation; breathing short for a considerable time; recovered his heat; thirst; passed the night quietly; slight sweats about the head. On the third, passed the day in a composed state; in the evening, about sunset, slight chills; nausea, agitation; passed the night in a painful state; had no sleep; small stools of compact faeces passed from the bowels. On the fourth, in the morning, composed; about noon all the symptoms became exacerbated; coldness, loss of speech, and of articulation; became worse; recovered his heat after a time; passed black urine, having substances floating in it; the night quiet; slept. On the fifth, seemed to be lightened, but a painful weight about the belly; thirsty, passed the night in a painful state. On the sixth, in the morning, in a quiet state; in the evening the pains greater; had a paroxysm; in the evening the bowels properly opened by a small clyster; slept at night. On the seventh, during the day, in a state of nausea, somewhat disturbed; passed urine of the appearance of oil; at night, much agitation, was incoherent, did not sleep. On the eighth, in the morning, slept a little; but immediately coldness, loss of speech, respiration small and weak; but in the evening recovered his heat again; was delirious, but towards day was somewhat lightened; stools small, bilious, and unmixed. On the ninth, affected with coma, and with nausea when roused; not very thirsty; about sunset he became restless and incoherent; passed a bad night. On the tenth, in the morning, had become speechless; great coldness; acute fever; much perspiration; he died. His sufferings were on the even days. Explanation of the characters. It is probable that the excessive sweats caused death on the tenth day.

CASE IV. The patient affected with phrenitis, having taken to bed on the first day, vomited largely of verdigris-green and thin matters; fever, accompanied with rigors, copious and continued sweats all over; heaviness of the head and neck, with pain; urine thin, substances floating in the urine small, scattered, did not subside; had copious dejections from the bowels; very delirious; no sleep. On the second, in the morning, loss of speech; acute fever; he sweated, fever did not leave him; palpitations over the whole body, at night, convulsions. On the third, all the symptoms exacerbated; he died. Explanation of the characters. It is probable that the sweats and convulsions caused death.

CASE V. In Larissa, a man, who was bald, suddenly was seized with pain in the right thigh; none of the things which were administered did him any good. On the first day, fever acute, of the ardent type, not agitated, but the pains persisted. On the second, the pains in the thigh abated, but the fever increased; somewhat tossed about; did not sleep; extremities cold; passed a large quantity of urine, not of a good character. On the third, the pain of the thigh ceased; derangement of the intellect, confusion, and much tossing about. On the fourth, about noon, he died. An acute disease.

CASE VI. In Abdera, Pericles was seized with a fever of the acute, continual type, with pain; much thirst, nausea, could not retain his drink; somewhat swelled about the spleen, with heaviness of the head. On the first day, had hemorrhage from the left nostril, but still the fever became more violent; passed much muddy, white urine, which when allowed to stand did not subside. On the second day, all the symptoms were exacerbated, yet the urine was thick, and more inclined to have a sediment; the nausea less; he slept. On the third, fever was milder; abundance of urine, which was concocted, and had a copious sediment; passed a quiet night. On the fourth, had a copious and warm sweat all over about noon; was free of fever, had a crisis, no relapse. An acute affection.

CASE VII. In Abdera, the young woman who was lodged in the Sacred Walk was seized with an ardent fever. She was thirsty, and could not sleep; had menstruation for the first time. On the sixth, much nausea, flushing, was chilly, and tossed about. On the seventh, in the same state; urine thin,but of a good color; no disturbance about the bowels. On the eighth, deafness, acute fever, insomnolency, nausea, rigors, became collected; urine the same. On the ninth, in the same state, and also on the following days; thus the deafness persisted. On the fourteenth, disorder of the intellect; the fever abated. On the seventeenth, a copious hemorrhage from the nose; the deafness slightly better; and on the following days, nausea, deafness, and incoherence. On the twentieth, pain of the feet; deafness and delirium left her; a small hemorrhage from the nose; sweat, apyrexia. On the twenty-fourth, the fever returned, deafness again; pain of the feet remained; incoherence. On the twenty-seventh, had a copious sweat, apyrexia; the deafness left her; the pain of her feet partly remained; in other respects had a complete crisis. Explanation of the characters. It is probable that the restoration of health on the twentieth day was the result of the evacuation of urine.

CASE VIII. In Abdera, Anaxion, who was lodged near the with Thracian Gates, was seized with an acute fever; pain of the right dry cough, without expectoration during the first days, thirst, insomnolency; urine well colored, copious, and thin. On the sixth, delirious; no relief from the warm applications. On the seventh, in a painful state, for the fever while the pains did not abate, and the cough was troublesome, and attended with dyspnoea. On the eighth, I opened a vein at the elbow, and much blood, of a proper character, flowed; the pains were abated, but the dry coughs continued. On the eleventh, the fever diminished; slight sweats about the head; coughs, with more liquid sputa; he was relieved. On the twentieth, sweat, apyrexia; but after the crisis he was thirsty, and the expectorations were not good. On the twenty-seventh the fever relapsed; he coughed, and brought up much concocted sputa: sediment in the urine copious and white; he became free of thirst, and the respiration was good. On the thirty-fourth, sweated all over, apyrexia general crisis. Explanation of the characters. It is probable that the evacuation of the sputa brought about the recovery on the thirty-fourth day.

CASE IX. In Abdera, Heropythus, while still on foot, had pain in the head, and not long afterwards he took to bed; he lived near the High Street. Was seized with acute fever of the ardent type; vomitings at first of much bilious matter; thirst; great restlessness; urine thin, black, substances sometimes floating high in it, and sometimes not; passed the night in a painful state; paroxysms of the fever diversified, and for the most part irregular. About the fourteenth day, deafness; the fever increased; urine the same. On the twentieth and following days, much delirium. On the thirtieth, copious hemorrhage from the nose, and became more collected; deafness continued, but less; the fever diminished; on the following days, frequent hemorrhages, at short intervals. About the sixtieth, the hemorrhages ceased, but violent pain of the hip-joint, and increase of fever. Not long afterwards, pains of all the inferior rule, that either the fever and deafness increased, or, pains of the inferior parts were increased. About the eightieth day, all the complaints gave way, without leaving any behind; for the urine was of a good color, and had a copious sediment, while the delirium became less. About the hundredth day, disorder of the bowels, with copious and bilious evacuations, and these continued for a considerable time, and again assumed the dysenteric form with pain; but relief of all the other complaints. On the whole, the fevers went off, and the deafness ceased. On the hundred and twentieth day, had a complete crisis. Ardent fever. Explanation of the characters. It is probable that the bilious discharge brought about the recovery on the hundred and twentieth day.

CASE X. In Abdera, Nicodemus was seized with fever from venery and drinking. At the commencement he was troubled with nausea and cardialgia; thirsty, tongue was parched; urine thin and dark. On the second day, the fever exacerbated; he was troubled with rigors and nausea; had no sleep; vomited yellow bile; urine the same; passed a quiet night, and slept. On the third, a general remission; amelioration; but about sunset felt again somewhat uncomfortable; passed an uneasy night. On the fourth, rigor, much fever, general pains; urine thin, with substances floating in it; again a quiet night. On the fifth, all the symptoms remained, but there was an amelioration. On the sixth, some general pains; substances floating in the urine; very incoherent. On the seventh, better. On the eighth, all the other symptoms abated. On the tenth, and following days, there were pains, but all less; in this case throughout, the paroxysms and pains were greater on the even days. On the twentieth, the urine white and thick, but when allowed to stand had no sediment; much sweat; seemed to be free from fever; but again in the evening he became hot, with the same pains, rigor, thirst, slightly incoherent. On the twenty-fourth, urine copious, white, with an abundant sediment; a copious and warm sweat all over; apyrexia; the fever came to its crisis. Explanation of the characters. It is probable that the cure was owing to the bilious evacuations and the sweats.

CASE XI. In Thasus, a woman, of a melancholic turn of mind, from some accidental cause of sorrow, while still going about, became affected with loss of sleep, aversion to food, and had thirst and nausea. She lived near the Pylates, upon the Plain. On the first, at the commencement of night, frights, much talking, despondency, slight fever; in the morning, frequent spasms, and when they ceased, she was incoherent and talked obscurely; pains frequent, great and continued. On the second, in the same state; had no sleep; fever more acute. On the third, the spasms left her; but coma, and disposition to sleep, and again awaked, started up, and could not contain herself; much incoherence; acute fever; on that night a copious sweat all over; apyrexia, slept, quite collected; had a crisis. About the third day, the urine black, thin, substances floating in it generally round, did not fall to the bottom; about the crisis a copious menstruation.

CASE XII. In Larissa, a young unmarried woman was seized with a fever of the acute and ardent type; insomnolency, thirst; tongue sooty and dry; urine of a good color, but thin. On the second, in an uneasy state, did not sleep. On the third, alvine discharges copious, watery, and greenish, and on the following days passed such with relief. On the fourth, passed a small quantity of thin urine, having substances floating towards its surface, which did not subside; was delirious towards night. On the sixth, a great hemorrhage from the nose; a chill, with a copious and hot sweat all over; apyrexia, had a crisis. In the fever, and when it had passed the crisis, the menses took place for the first time, for she was a young woman. Throughout she was oppressed with nausea, and rigors; redness of the face; pain of the eyes; heaviness of the head; she had no relapse, but the fever came to a crisis. The pains were on the even days.

CASE XIII. Apollonius, in Abdera, bore up (under the fever?) for some time, without betaking himself to bed. His viscera were enlarged, and for a considerable time there was a constant pain about the liver, and then he became affected with jaundice; he was flatulent, and of a whitish complexion. Having eaten beef, and drunk unseasonably, he became a little heated at first, and betook himself to bed, and having used large quantities of milk, that of goats and sheep, and both boiled and raw, with a bad diet otherwise, great mischief was occasioned by all these things; for the fever was exacerbated, and of the food taken scarcely any portion worth mentioning was passed from the bowels; the urine was thin and scanty; no sleep; troublesome meteorism; much thirst; disposition to coma; painful swelling of the right hypochondrium; extremities altogether coldish; slight incoherence, forgetfulness of everything he said; he was beside himself. About the fourteenth day after he betook himself to bed, had a rigor, became heated, and was seized with furious delirium; loud cries, much talking, again composed, and then coma came on; afterwards the bowels disordered, with copious, bilious, unmixed, and undigested stools; urine black, scanty, and thin; much restlessness; alvine evacuations of varied characters, either black, scanty, and verdigrisgreen, or fatty, undigested, and acrid; and at times the dejections resembled milk. About the twenty-fourth, enjoyed a calm; other matters in the same state; became somewhat collected; remembered nothing that had happened since he was confined to bed; immediately afterwards became delirious; every symptom rapidly getting worn. About the thirtieth, acute fever; stools copious and thin; was delirious; extremities cold; loss of speech. On the thirty-fourth he died. In this case, as far as I saw, the bowels were disordered; urine thin and black; disposition to coma; insomnolency; extremities cold; delirious throughout. Phrenitis.

CASE XIV. In Cyzicus, a woman who had brought forth twin daughters, after a difficult labor, and in whom the lochial discharge was insufficient, at first was seized with an acute fever, attended with chills; heaviness of the head and neck, with pain; insomnolency from the commencement; she was silent, sullen, and disobedient; urine thin, and devoid of color; thirst, nausea for the most part; bowels irregularly disordered, and again constipated. On the sixth, towards night, talked much incoherently; had no sleep. About the eleventh day was seized with wild delirium, and again became collected; urine black, thin, and again deficient, and of an oily appearance; copious, thin, and disordered evacuations from the bowels. On the fourteenth, frequent convulsions;extremities cold; not in anywise collected; suppression of urine. On the sixteenth loss of speech. On the seventeenth, she died. Phrenitis. Explanation of the characters. It is probable that death was caused, on the seventeenth day, by the affection of the brain consequent upon her accouchement.

CASE XV. In Thasus, the wife of Dealces, who was lodged upon the Plain, from sorrow was seized with an acute fever, attended with chills. From first to last she wrapped herself up in her bedclothes; still silent, she fumbled, picked, bored, and gathered hairs (from them); tears, and again laughter; no sleep; bowels irritable, but passed nothing; when directed, drank a little; urine thin and scanty; to the touch of the hand the fever was slight; coldness of the extremities. On the ninth, talked much incoherently, and again became composed and silent. On the fourteenth, breathing rare, large, at intervals; and again hurried respiration. On the sixteenth, looseness of the bowels from a stimulant clyster; afterwards she passed her drink, nor could retain anything, for she was completely insensible; skin parched and tense. On the twentieth, much talk, and again became composed; loss of speech; respiration hurried. On the twenty-first she died. Her respiration throughout was rare and large; she was totally insensible; always wrapped up in her bedclothes; either much talk, or completely silent throughout. Phrenitis.

CASE XVI. In Meliboea, a young man having become heated by drinking and much venery, was confined to bed; he was affected with rigors and nausea; insomnolency and absence of thirst. On the first day much faeces passed from the bowels along with a copious flux; and on the following days he passed many watery stools of a green color; urine thin, scanty, and deficient in color; respiration rare, large, at long intervals; softish distention of the hypochondrium, of an oblong form, on both sides; continued palpitation in the epigastric region throughout; passed urine of an oily appearance. On the tenth, he had calm delirium, for he was naturally of an orderly and quiet disposition; skin parched and tense; dejections either copious and thin, or bilious and fatty. On the fourteenth, all the symptoms were exacerbated; he became delirious, and talked much incoherently. On the twentieth, wild delirium, On the twentieth, wild delirium, jactitation, passed no urine; small drinks were retained. On the twenty-fourth he died. Phrenitis.

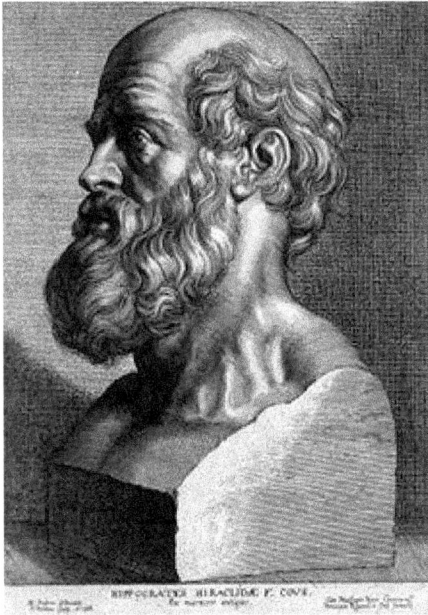

HIPPO'CRATES, the second of that name, and in some respects the most celebrated physician of ancient or modern times ; for not only have his writings (or rather those which bear his name) been always held in the highest esteem, but his personal history (so far as it is known), and the literary criticism relating to his works, furnish so much matter for the consideration both of the scholar, the philologist, the philosopher, and the man of letters, that there are few authors of antiquity about whom so much has been written.

Probably the readers of this work will care more for the literary than for the medical questions connected with Hippocrates ; and accordingly (as it is quite impossible to discuss the whole subject fully in these pages) the strictly scientific portion of this article occupies less space than the critical ; and this arrangement in this place the writer is inclined to adopt the more readily, because, while there are many works which contain a good account of the scientific merits of the Hippocratic writings, he is not aware of one where the many literary problems arising from them have been at once fully discussed and satisfactorily determined. This task he is far from thinking that he has himself accomplished, but it is right to give this reason for treating the scientific part of the subject much less fully than he would have done had he been writing for a professed medical work.

A parallel has more than once been drawn be- tween " the Father of Medicine " and " the Father of Poetry ; " and, indeed, the resemblances between the two, both in their personal and literary historj', are so evident, that they could hardly fail to strike any one who was even moderately familiar with classical and medical literature. With respect to their personal history, the greatest uncertainty exists, and our real knowledge is next to nothing ; although in the case of both personages, we have professed lives written by ancient authors, which, however, only tend to show still more plainly the ignorance that prevails on the subject. Accordingly, as might be expected, fable has been busy in supplying the deficiencies of history, and was for a time fully believed ; till •sX length a re-action fol- lowed, and an unreasoning credulity was succeeded by an equally unreasonable scepticism, which reached its climax when it was boldly asserted that neither Homer nor Hippocrates had ever ex- istfid. (See Ilouclart, Etudes sur IJifypocrate^ p. 6G0.) The few facts respecting him that may be considered as tolerably well ascertained may be told in few words. His father was Ileracleides, who was also a physician, and belonged to the family of the Asclepiadae. According to Soraniis (Vita Hippocr.^ in Ilippocr. Opera, vol. iii.), he was the nineteenth in descent from Aesculapius, but John Tzetzes, who gives the genealogy of the family, makes him the seventeenth. His niotlier's name was Phaenarete, who was said to be descended from Hercules. Soranus, on tlie autho- rity of an old writer who had composed a life of Hippocrates, states that he was born in the island of Cos, in the first year of the eightieth Olympiad, that is. B. c. 460 ; and this date is generally followed, for want of any more satisfactory inform- ation on the subject, though it agrees so ill with some of the anecdotes respecting him, that some persons suppose hira to have been born about thirty years sooner. The exact day of his birth was known and celebrated in Cos with sacrifices on the '26th. day of the month Agrianus,but it is unknown to what date in any other calendar this month cor- responds. He was instructed in medical science by his father and by Herodicus, and is also said to have been a pupil of Gorgias of Leontini. He wrote, taught, and practised his profession at home ; travelled in different parts of the continent of Greece ; and died at Larissa in Thessaly. His age at the time of his death is uncertain, as it is stated by different ancient authors to have been eighty-five years, ninety, one hundred and four, fend one hundred and nine. Mr. Clinton places his death B. c. 357, at the age of one hundred and four. He had two sons, Thessalus and Dracon, and a son-in-law, Polybus, all of whom followed the same profession, and who are supposed to have been the authors of some of the works in the Hippocratic Collection. Such are the few and scanty facts that can be in some degree depended on respecting the personal history of this cele- brated man ; but though we have not the means of writing an authentic detailed biography, we possess in these few facts, and in the hints and allusions con- tained in various ancient authors, sufficient data to enable us to appreciate the part he played, and the place he held among his contemporaries. We find that he enjoyed their esteem as a practitioner, writer, and professor; that he conferred on the ancient and illustrious family to which he belonged more honour than he derived from it ; that he rendered the medical school of Cos, to which he was attached, superior to any which had preceded it or immediately followed it ; and that his works, soon after their publication, were studied and quoted by Plato. (See Littre's Hippocr. vol. i. p. 43 ; and a review of that work (by the writer of this article) in the Brit, and For. Med. Rev. April, 1844, p. 459.)

Upon this slight foundation of historical truth has been built a vast superstructure of fabulous error ; and it is curious to observe how all these tales receive a colouring from the times and coun- tries in which they appear to have been fabricated, whether by his own countrymen before the Chris- tian era, or by the Latin or Arabic writers of the middle ages. One of the stories told of him by his Greek biograpners, which most modern critics are disposed to regard as fabulous, relates to his being sent for, together with Euryphon [EuRV- phon], by Perdiccas II., king of Macedonia, and discovering, by certain external symptoms, that his sickness was occasioned by his having fallen in love with his father's concubine. Probably the strongest reason against the truth of this story is the fact that the time of the supposed cure is quite irreconcileable with the commonly received date of the birth of Hippocrates ; though M. Litire, the latest and best editor of Hippocrates, while he rejects the story as spurious, finds no difficulty in the dates (vol. i. p. 38). Soranus, who tells tlie anecdote, says that the occurrence took place after the death of Alexander I., the father of Perdiccas; and we may rcasonabl} *presume that one or two* years would be the longest interval that would elapse. The date of the death of Alexander is not exactly known, and depends upon the length of the reign of his son Perdiccas, who died b. c. 414. The longest period assigned to his reign is forty- one years, the shortest is twenty-three. This latter date would place his accession to the throne on his father's death, at B. c. 437, at which time Hippo- crates would be only twenty-three years old, almost too young an age for him to have acquired so great celebrity as to be specially sent for to attend a foreign prince. However, the date of B. c. 437 is the less probable because it would not only extend the reign of his father Alexander to more than sixty years, but would also suppose him to have lived seventy years after a period at which he was already grown up to manhood. For these reasons Mr. Clinton {F. Hell. ii. 222) agrees with Dodwell in supposing the longer periods assigned to his reign to be nearer the truth ; and assumes the ac- cession of Perdiccas to have fallen within B. c. 454, at which time Hippocrates was only six years old. This celebrated story has been told, with more or less variation, of Erasistratus and Avicenna, besides being interwoven in the romance of Heliodorus (Aet/dop. iv, 7. p. 171), and the love-letters of Aristaenetus (Epist. i. 13). Galen also says that a similar circumstance happened to himself. (De Praenot. ad Epig. c. 6. vol. xiv. p. 630.) The story as applied to Avicenna seems to be most probably apocryphal (see Biogr. Diet, of the Usef. Knowl. Soc. vol. iv. p. 301) ; and with respect to the two other claimants, Hippocrates and Erasistratus, if it be true of either, the pre- ponderance of historical testimony is decidedly in favour of the latter. [Erasistratus.] Another old Greek fable relates to his being appointed librarian at Cos, and burning the books there (or, according to another version of the story, at Cnidos,) in order to conceal the use he had made of them in his own writings. This story is also told, with but little variation, of Avicenna, and is repeated of Hippocrates, with some characteristic embellish- ments, in the European Legends of the Middle Ages. [Andrkas.]

The other fables concerning Hippocrates are to be traced to the collection of Letters, &c. which go under his name, but which are universally rejected as spurious. The most celebrated of these relates to his supposed conduct during the plague of Athens, which he is said to have stopped by burn- ing fires throughout the city, by suspending chap- lets of flowers, and by the use of an antidote, the composition of which is preserved by Joannes Ac- tuarius {De Meth. Med. v. 6. p. 264, ed. H. Steph.) Connected with this, is the pretended letter from Artaxerxes Longimanus, king of Persia, to Hippocrates, inviting him by great offers to come to his assistance during a time of pestilence, and the re- fusal of Hippocrates, on the ground of his being the enemy of his country.

Another story, perhaps equally familiar to the readers of Burton's "Anatomy of Melancholy," contains the history of the supposed madness of Democritus, and his interview with Hippocrates, who had been sunnnoned by his countrymen to come to his relief.

If we turn to the Arabic writers, we find " Bokrdt " represented as living at Hems, and studying in a garden near Damascus, the situation of which was still pointed out in the time of Abu-1- faraj in the thirteenth century. (Abu-1-faraj, Hist. Dynast, p. 56; Anon. Arab.

Philosoph. Bibl. apud Casiri, Bihlioth. A rahico-Hisp. Escur. vol. i. p. 235.) They also tell a story of his pupils taking his por- trait to a celebrated physiognomist named Phile- mon., in order to try his skill ; and that upon his saying that it was the portrait of a lascivious old man (which they strenuously denied), Hippocrates said that he was right, for that he was so by nature, but that he had learned to overcome his amorous propensities. The confusion of names that occurs in this last anecdote the writer has never seen explained, though the difficulty admits of an easy and satisfactory solution. It will no doubt have brought to the reader's recollection the similar story told of Socrates by Cicero (Tusc. Disp. iv. 37, De Fata., c. 5), and accordingly he will be quite prepared to hear that the Arabic writers have confounded the word]b^ JL«j Sokrut^ with ^^ Jj Boki-at., and have thus applied to Hippocrates an anecdote that in reality belongs to Socrates. The name of the physiognomist in Cicero is Zopyrus, which cannot have been corrupted into Philemon ; but when we remember that the Arabians have no /*, and are therefore often obliged to express this letter by an F^ it will probably appear not unlikely that either the writers, or their European trans- lators, have confounded Philemon with Polemon. This conjecture is confirmed by the fact that Phile- mon is said by Abu-1-faraj to have written a work on Physiognomy, which is true of Polemon, whose treatise on that subject is still extant, whereas no person of the name of Philemon (as far as the writer is aware) is mentioned as a physiognomist by any Greek author.* The only objection to this conjecture is the anachronism of making Pole- mon a contemporary of Hippocrates or Socrates ; but this difficulty will not appear very great to any one who is familiar with the extreme igno- rance and carelessness displayed by the Arabic writers on all points of Greek history and chro- nology.

It is, however, among the European story- tellers of the middle ages that the name of " Ypo- cras " is most celebrated. In one story he is repre- sented as visiting Rome during the reign of Au- gustus, and restoring to life the emperor's nephew, who was just dead ; for which service Augustus

- There is at this present time among the MSS.

at Leyden a little Arabic treatise on Physiognomy which bears the name of Philemon., and which (as the writer has been informed by a gentleman who has compared the two works) bears a very great resemblance to the Greek treatise by Polemon. {JXQ Catal. Biblioth. Lujdun. p. 461. § 1286.)

erected a statue in his honour as to a divinity. A fair lady resolved to prove that this god was a mere mortal ; and, accordingly, having made an assignation with him, she let down for him a basket from her window. When she had raised him half way, she left him suspended in the air all night, till he was found by the emperor in the morning, and thus became the laughing-stock of the court. Anoiher story makes him professor of medicine in Rome, with a nephew of wondrous talents and medical skill, whom he despatched in his own stead to the king of Hungary, who had sent for him to heal his son. The young leech, by his marvellous skill, having discovered that the prince was not the king's own son, directed him to feed on " contrarius drink, contrarius mete, beves flesch, and drink the broth t," and thereby soon restored him to health. Upon his return home laden with presents, " Ypocras" became so jealous of his fame, that he murdered him, and afterwards " he let all his bokes berne." The vengeance of Heaven overtook him, and he died in dreadful torments, confessing his crime, and vainly calling on his murdered nephew for relief. (See Ellis, Spec, of Early Engl. Metr. Roman, vol. iii. p. 39 ; Weber, Metr. Rom. of the Wi, Uh, and bth Cent.., ^c, vol. iii. p. 41 ; Way, Fabliaux or Talcs of the ih and 'Mh Cent.^ ^c. vol. ii. p. 173 ; Le- grand d'Aussy, Fabliaux ou Contes, Fables et Ro- mans du eme et du ?>eme Siecles, tome i. p. 288 ; Loiseleur Deslongchamps, Essai sur les Fables Ind. ^c, p. 154, and Roman des Sept Sages, p. 26.)

If, from the personal history of Hippocrates, we turn to the collection of writings that go under his name, the parallel with Homer will be still more exact and striking. In both cases we find a number of works, the most ancient, and, in some respects, the most excellent of their kind, which, though they have for centuries borne the same name, are discovered, on the most cursory examination, to belong in reality to several different persons. Hence has arisen a question which has for ages exercised the learning and acuteness of scholars and critics, and which is in both cases still far from being satisfactorily settled. With respect to the writings of the Hippocratic Collection " the first glance," says M. Littre (vol. i. p. 44), *' shows that some are complete in themselves, while others are merely collections of notes, which follow each other without connection, and which are sometimes hardly intelligible. Some are incomplete and fragmentary, others form in the whole Collection particular series, which belong to the same ideas and the same writer. In a word, however little we reflect ou the context of these numerous writings, we are led to conclude that they are not the work of one and the same author. This remark has in all ages struck those persons who have given their atten- tion to the works of Hippocrates ; and even at the time when men commented on them in the Alex- andrian school, they already disputed about their authenticity."

But it is not merely from internal evidence (though this of itself would be sufficiently con- vincing) that we find that the Hippocratic Collec- tion is not the work of Hippocrates alone, for it so happens that in two insUinces we find a passage that has appeared from very early times as forming part of this collection, quoted as belonging to a dilfereut person. Indeed if we had nothing but internal evidence to guide us in our task of ex- amining these writings, in order to decide which really belong to Hippocrates, we should come to but few positive results ; and therefore it is neces- sary to collect all the ancient testimonies that can still be found ; in doing which, it will appear that the Collection, as a whole, can be traced no higher than the period of the Alexandrian school, in the third century b. c. ; but that particular treatises are referred to by the contemporaries of Hippocrates and his immediate successors. {^Brit. and For. Med. Rev. p. 460.)

We find that Hippocrates is mentioned or re- ferred to by no less than ten persons anterior to the foundation of the Alexandrian school, and among them by Aristotle and Plato. At the time of the formation of the great Alexandrian library, the different treatises which bear the name of Hip- pocrates were diligently sought for, and formed into a single collection ; and about this time commences the series of Commentators, which has continued through a period of more than two thousand years to the present day. The first person who is known to have commented on any of the works of the Hippocratic Collection is Herophilus. [Herophi- Lus.] The most ancient commentary still in ex- istence is that on the treatise " De Articulis," by ApoUonius Citiensis. [Apollonius Citiensis.] By far the most voluminous, and at the same time by far the most valuable commentaries that remain, are those of Galen, who wrote several works in illustration of the writings of Hippocrates, besides those which we now possess. His Commentaries, which are still extant, are those on the " De Na- tura Hominis," " De Salubri Victus Ratione," " De Ratione Victus in Morbis Acutis," " Praenotiones," " Praedictiones I.," " Aphorismi," " De Morbis Vulgaribus I. II. III. VI," " De Fracturis," "De Articulis," " De OfRcina Medici," and " De Hu- moribus," with a glossary of difficult and obsolete words, and fragments on the " De Aere, Aquis, et Locis," and " De Alimento." The other ancient commentaries that remain are those of Palladius, Joannes Alexandrinus, Stephanus Atheniensis, Meletius, Theophilus Protospatharius, and Damas- cius ; besides a spurious work attributed to Ori- basius, a glossary of obsolete and difficult words by I'lrotianus, and some Arabic Commentaries that have never been published. {^Brit. and For. Med. Rev. p. 461.)

His writings were held in the highest esteem by the ancient Greek and Latin physicians, and most of them were translated into Arabic. (See Wen- rich, De Auct. Grace. Vers, et Comment. Syr. Arab., &c.) In the middle ages, however, they were not so much studied as those of some other authors, whose works are of a more practical cha- racter, and better fitted for being made a class-book and manual of instruction. In more modern times, on the contrary, the works of the Hippocratic Col- lection have been valued more according to their real worth, while many of the most popular medical writers of the middle ages have fallen into complete neglect. The number of works written in illustra- tion or explanation of the Collection is very great, as is also that of the editions of the whole or any part ol the treatises composing it. Of these only a very few can be here mentioned : a fuller account may be found in Fabric. Bibl. Grace. ; Haller, Bibl. Medic. Pract.; the first vol. of Kiihn's edi- tion of Hippocrates; Choulanfs Ilandb. der Bu- clierTcunde fur die Aellere Medicin ; Littre's Hip- pocrates ; and other professed bibliographical works. 'J'he works of Hippocrates first appeared in a Latin translation by Fabius Calvus, Rom. 1525, fol. The first Greek edition is the Aldine, Venet. 1526, fol., which was printed from MSS. with hardly any correction of the transcriber's errors. The first edition that had any pretensions to be called a critical edition was that by Hieron. Mercurialis, Venet. 1588, fol., Gr. and Lat. ; but this was much surpassed by that of Anut. Foesius, Francof. 1595, fol., Gr. and Lat., which continues to the present day to be the best complete edition. Van- der Linden's edition (Lugd. Bat. 1 665, 8vo. 2 vols. Gr. and Lat.) is neat and commodious for refer- ence from his having divided the text into short paragraphs. Chartier's edition of the works of Galen and Hippocrates has been noticed under Galen; as has also Kiihn's, of which it may be said that its only advantages are its convenient size, the reprint of Ackermann's Histor. Liter. Hippocr. (from Harless's ed. of Fabr. Bibl. Gr.) in the first vol., and the noticing on each page the cor- responding pagination of the editions of Foes, Chartier, and Vander Linden. By far the best edition in every respect is one which is now in the course of publication at Paris, under the super- intendence of E. Littre, of which the first vol. ap- peared in 1839, and the fourth in 1844. It contains a new text, founded upon a collation of the MSS. in the Royal Library at Paris ; a French translation ; an interesting and learned general In- troduction, and a copious argument prefixed to each treatise ; and numerous scientific and philological notes. It is a work quite indispensable to every physician, critic, and philologist, who wishes to study in detail the works of the Hippocratic Col- lection, and it has already done much more to- wards settling the text than any edition that has preceded it ; but at the same time it must not be concealed that the editor does not seem to have always made the best use of the materials that he has had at his command, and that the classical reader cannot help now and then noticing a mani- fest want of critical (and even at times of gram- matical) scholarship.

The Hippocratic Collection consists of more than sixty works ; and the classification of these, and assigning each (as far as possible) to its proper author, constitutes by far the most diffi- cult question connected with the ancient medical writers. Various have been the classifications proposed both in ancient and modem times, and various the rules by which their authors were guided ; some contenting themselves with following implicitly the opinions of Galen and Erotianus, others arguing chiefly from peculiarities of style, while a tliird class distinguished the books accord- ing to the medical and philosophical doctrines contained in them. An account of each of these classifications cannot be given here, much less can the objections that may be brought against each be pointed out : upon the whole, the writer is inclined to think M. Littre's superior to any that has pre- ceded it ; but by no means so imexceptionable as to do away with the necessity of a new one. The following classification, though far enough from supplying the desideratum, difi'ers in several in- stances from any former one : it is impossible here for the writer to give more than the results of his investigation, referring for the data on which hia opinion in each particular case is founded to the works of Gniner, Ackermann, and Littre, of which he has, of course, made free use.* Perhaps a tabular or genealogical view of the different divisions and subdivisions of the Collection will be the best cal- culated to put the reader at once in possession of the whole bearings of the subject.

The Hippocratic Collection consists of Works certainltf ■written by Hip- pocrates. (Class Works certainly not written by Hippocrates. Works perhaps written by Hip- pocrates. (Class ll.) Works earliei than Hippo- crates. (Class III.) Works later than Hippo- crates. Works about contemporary with Hippo- crates. I >Vorks authentic, but not genuine, i. e. not wilful forgeries. Works neither genuine nor authentic, i.e. wilful forge- ries. (Class VIII.) I I Works whose Works whose author is author is conjectured. unknown. (Class IV.) (Class V.) Works by va- rious authors. (Class VII.) Works by the same author. (Class VI.)

Class I., containing UpoyuaxTTiKdv, Praenotiones or Prognosticon (vol. i. p. 88, ed. Kiihn) ; 'A^o- pia-fiol, Aphorismi (vol. iii. p. 706) ; 'EiridTjixicou Bi§ia A, r, De Morbis Popularilms (or Epidemi- orum lib. i. and iii. (vol. i. pp. 382, 467) ; Hept AjaiTTjs 'O | 6ojj', De Ratione Victus in Morbis Acutis, or De Diaeta Acutorum (vol. ii. p. 25); Tlepi *Aepiou^ 'TSdruv^ Tottwv, De Acre, Aquisy et Locis (vol. i. p, 523) ; Uepl twu kv KecpoKfj Tpu- ixdruu, De Capitis Vulneribus (vol. iii. p. 346).

Class II., containing Ilepl "Apxaf-ns 'iTjTpj/crjy, De Prisca Medidna (vol. i. p. 22) ; Hep! "Apdpwv, De Articidis (vol. iii. p. 135); Uepl ^KyixSv^ De Fradis (vol. iii. p. 64); MoxA.tKos, MochUms or Vectiarius (vol. iii. p. 270) ; "OpKos, Jicsjurandum (vol. i. p. 1) ; ^o/xos. Lex (vol. i. p. 3); Ilepl 'E/c(Sj', De Ulceribus (vol. iii. p. 307) ; Tl^pX ^vpiyywv^ De Fistulis (vol. iii. p. 329); Uepl AtfjLo^pot^cov^ De Haemorrhoidibus (o. iii. p. 340); KaT* 'iTjrpetoj', De Officina Medici (vol. iii. p. 48) ; TlepX 'Iprjs Uovaov^ De Morbo Sacra (vol. i. p. 587).

Class III., containing Tlpo^f)7}riK6v A, Pror- rlietica^ or Praedidiones i. (vol. i. p. 157) ; KcoaKot npoyvdaeis, Coacae Praenotiones (vol. i. p. 234).

Class IV., containing Uspl ^vcrios 'Avdpciirov, De Natura Hominis (vol. i. p. 348) ; riepl Aiairrts "Tyieivrjs, De Salubri Victus Ratione {?)

(vol. i. p. 616); riepl TouaiK^i-n^ ^uaios, De Natura Mu- liebri(?) (vol. ii. p. 529) ; Uepl Nomwv B, T, De Morbis, ii. iii(?) (volii. p.212); Uepl 'EmKv^<rios, De Super/oetatione{?) (vol. i. p. 460).

Class v., containing Uepl Ouawi', De Phtibus (vol. i. p. 569) ; Uepl TSituv twv kut "AvOpwrrov^ De Locis in Homine (vol. ii. p. 101) ; Ilepl Texi'Tjy, De Arte{?) (vol. i. p. 5) ; Uepl AiatTijs, De Diaeta, or De Victus Ratione (vol. i. p. 625) ; Uepl 'Ei/u-

- Some of the readers of this work may perhaps

be interested to hear that a strictly ;)A«7o/or/2ca/ clas- sification of the works of the Hippocratic Collection is still a desideratum ; and that, as this is in fact almost the only question connected with the subject which has not by this time been thoroughly ex- amined, any scholar who will undertake the work will be doing good service to the cause of ancient medical literature.

■npltav, De Insomniis (vol. ii. p. 1); Uepl UaOwv, De Affectionibus (vol. ii. p. 380) ; Uepl tcov evros UadoSu, De Internis Affectionilms (vol. ii. p. 427) ; Uepl Novaav A, De Morbis i. (vol. ii. p. 1 65) ; Uepl 'EirTajj-riuov, De Septimestri Partu (vol. i. p. 444) ; Uepl 'OKTafxrivov, De Octimestri Partu (vol. i. p. 455) ; ^EiTi8'r]ixi(av Bi§la B, A, Z, Epidemiorum, or De Morbis Popularibtis, ii. iv. vi. (vol. iii. pp. 428, 511, 583) ; Uepl Xv/jlu/v, De Ilumoribus (vol. i. p. 120) ; Uepl 'Typwv Xpijaios, De Usu Liqui- dorum (vol. ii. p. 153).

Class VI., containing Uepl Vovrs, De Genitura (vol. i. p. 371) ; Uepl ^va-ios UaiSiov, De Natura Pueri (vol. i. p. 382) ; Ilepl 'No^awv A, De Morbis iv. (vol. ii. p. 324) ; Uepl TuvaiKeim', De Mu- lierum Morbis (vol. ii. p. 606) ; Utpl Uap6ei>iw}/, De Virginum Morbis (vol. ii. p. 526) ; Uepl 'A(p6- puiv, De Sterilibus (vol. iii. p. 1).

Class VII., containing 'EttjStJjUiwi' BigAta E, H, Epidemiorum, or De Morbis Popularibus v. vii. fvol. iii. pp. 545, 631) ; UeX KapStTjy, De Corde (vol. i. p. 485) ; Ilept Tpo<pT/s, De Alimento (vol. ii. p. 17) ; Ilept ^dpKoou, De Carnibus (vol. i. p. 424); Uepl 'ESSofjidSuv, De Septimanis, a work which no longer exists in Greek, but of which M. Littr6 has found a Latin translation ; Upop^rjTiKou B, Prorrhetica (or Praedidiones) ii. (vol. i. p. 185) ; Uepl 'Oa-Tewu ^vcrios, De Natura Ossium, a work composed entirely of extracts from other treatises of

the Hippocratic Collection, and from other an- cient authors, and which therefore M. Littre is going to suppress entirely (vol. i. p. 502) ; Uepl 'ASevwu, De Glandtdis (vol. i. p. 491); Uepl 'iTjTpov, De Medico (vol. i. p. 56) ; Uepl Ev- o'XVfJ-oavvTjs, De Decenti Habitu (vol. i. p. 66) ; UapayyeXiai, Praeceptiones (vol. i. p. 77) ; Uepl 'AvaTopLris, De Anatomia (or De Resedione Cor- porum) (vol. iii. p. 379) ; Uepl 'OSourocpvi'-ns, De Dmtitione (vol. i. p. 482) ; Uepl ^Ey Kararojxris 'E/i- Spvov, De Resedione Foetus (vol. iii. p. 376) ; Uepl "Oxl/ios, De Visu (vol. iii. p. 42) ; Uepl Kpialcau, De Crisibus (or De Judicationibus) (vol. i. p. 136) ; Uepl Kpiaifxwu, De Diebus Criticis (or De Diebus Judicatortis) (vol. i. p. 149) ; Uepl ^apixoLKoav, De Medicamentis Purgativis (vol. iii. p. 855 j.

Class VIII., containing 'EtnaroKal, Epistolae (vol. iii. p. 769) ; UpecrSevrinos ©eaaaXou, Tlies- sali Legati Oratio (vol. iii. p. 831); 'Etv iSoifxios, Oratio ad Aram (vol. iii. p. 830) ; Aoyjxa 'AOrj- vaicov, Atlieniensium Senatus Consultum (vol. iii. p. 829).

Each of these classes requires a few words of explanation. The first class will probably be con- sidered by many persons to be rather small ; but it seemed safer and better to include in it only those works of whose genuineness there has never been any doubt. To this there is perhaps one ex- ception, and that relating to the very work whose genuineness one would perhaps least expect to find called in question, as it is certainly that by which Hippocrates is most popularly known. Some doubts have arisen in the minds of several eminent critics as to the origin of the Aphorisms, and indeed the discussion of the genuineness of this work may be said to be an epitome of the questions relating to the whole Hippocratic Collection. We find here a very celebrated work, which has from early times borne the name of Hippocrates, but of which some parts have always been condemned as spurious. Upon examining tliose portions that are considered to be genuine, we observe that the greater part of the first three sections agrees almost word for word with passages to be found in his acknowledged works ; while in the remaining sections we find sentences fciken apparently from spurious or doubt- ful treatises ; thus adding greatly to our difficulties, inasmuch as they sometimes contain doctrines and theories opposed to those which we find in the works acknowledged to be genuine. And these facts are (in the opinion of the critics alluded to) to be accounted for in one of two ways : either

Hippocrates himself in his old age (for the Apho- risms have always been attributed to this period of his life) put together certain extracts from his own works, to which were afterwards added other sen- tences taken from later authors ; or else the col- lection was not formed by Hippocrates himself, but by some person or persons after his death, who made aphoristical extracts from his works, and from those of other writers of a later date, and the whole was then attributed to Hippocrates, because he was the author of the sentences that were most valuable, and came first in order. This account of the formation of the Aphorisms appears extremely plausible, nor does it seem to be any decisive ob- jection to say, that we find among them sentences which are not to be met with elsewhere ; for, when we recollect how many works of the old medical writers, and perhaps of Hippocrates himself, are lost, it is easy to conceive that these sentences may have been extracted from some treatise that is no longer in existence. It must however be con- fessed that this conjecture, however plausible and probable, requires further proof and examination before it can be received as true.

The second class is one of the most unsatisfac- tory in the writers own opinion, and affords at the same time a curious instance of the impossibility of satisfying even those few persons in Europe whose opinion on such a matter is really worth asking ; fi)r, upon submitting the classification to two friends, one of whom is decidedly the most learned phy- sician in Great Britain, and the other one of the best medical critics on the continent, he was ad- vised by the one to call this class "Works probably written by Hippocrates," and by the other to trans- fer them (with one exception) to the class of

- ' Works certainly not written by Hippocrates."

The amount of probability in favour of the genuine- ness of all these works is certainly by no means equal ; e. g. the two little pieces called the " Oath," and thS " Law," though commonly considered to be the work of the same author, and to be in- timately connected with each other, seem rather to belong to different periods, the former having all the simplicity, honesty, and religious feeling of an- tiquity, the latter somewhat of the affectation and declamatory grandiloquence of a sophist. How- ever, as all of these books have been considered to be genuine by some critics of more or less note, it seemed better to defer to their authority at least 80 far as to allow that they might perhaps have been written by Hippocrates himself.

The two works which constitute the third class, and which are probably the oldest medical writings that exist, have been supposed with some proba- bility to consist, at least in part, of the inscriptions on the votive tablets placed in the temple of Aescu- lapius by those who had recovered their health, which certJiinly constituted one of the sources from which the medical knowledge of Hippocrates was derived.

In the fourth class are placed those works which were certainly not written by Hippocrates himself, which were probably either contemporary or but little posterior to him, and whose authors have been, with more or less degree of certainty, dis- covered. The works De Natura Hoini/ns, and I)e Salubri Victus Ratmie^ are supposed by M. Littre to have been written by the same author, because it is said by Galen that in many old editions these two treatises formed but one ; and this author he concludes to have been Polybus, the son-in-law of Hippocrates (vol. i. pp. 46, 316, &c.), because a passage is quoted by Aristotle {Hist. Aiiiin. .iii ?>), and attributed to Polybus, which is found word for word in the work De Natura Iluminis (vol. i. p. 364). For somewhat similar reasons, Euryphon has been supposed to be the author of the second and third books De Morbis, and the work De Natura Muliebri [Euryphon] ; and also (though with much less show of reason) a certain Leo- phanes, or Cleophanes (of whom nothing whatever is known), to have written the treatise De Sujxrr- foetatione (Littr^, vol. i p. 380).

In the fifth class there is one treatise {De Di- aeta) in which an astronomical, coincidence with the calendar of Eudoxus has been pointed to the writer by a friend, which (as far as he is aware) has never been noticed by any commentator on Hippocrates, and which seems in some degree to fix the date of the work in question. If the ca- lendar of Eudoxus, as preserved in the Ajyparentiae of Ptolemy and the calendar of Geminus (see Petav. Uranol. pp. 64, 71), be compared with part of the third book De Diaeta (vol. i. pp. 7 1 1 —7 1 5), it will be found that the periods correspond so exactly, that (there being no other solar calendar of antiquity in which these intervals coincide so closely,and all through,but that of Eudoxus), it seems a reasonable inference that the writer of the work De Diaeta took them from the calendar in question. If this be granted, it will follow that the author must have written this work after the year B. c. 381, which is the date of the calendar of Eu- doxus ; and, as Hippocrates must have been at least eighty years old at that time, this conclusion will agree quite well with the general opinion of ancient and modern critics, that the treatise in question was probably written by one of his im- mediate followers.

The sixth class agrees with the sixth class of M. Littr^, who, with great appearance of proba- bility, supposes it to form a connected series of works written by the same author, whose name is quite unknown, and of whose date it can only be determined from internal evidence that he must have lived later than Hippocrates, and before the time of Aristotle.

The works contained in this and the seventh class have for many centuries formed part of the Hippocratic Collection without having any right to such an honour, and therefore are not genuine ; but, as it does not appear that their authors were guilty of assuming the name of Hippocrates, or that they have represented the state of medical science as in any respect different from what it really was in the times in which they wrote, there is no reason for denying their authenticity. And in this respect they are to be regarded with a very different eye from the pieces which form the last class, which are neither genuine nor authentic, but mere forgeries ; which display indeed here and there some ingenuity and skill, but which are still sufficiently full of difficulties and inconsistencies to betray at once their origin.

So much space has been taken up with the pre- liminary, but most indispensable step of determin- ing which are the genuine works of Hippocrates, and which are spurious, that a very slight sketch of his opinions is all that can be now attempted, and for a fuller account the reader must be referred to the works of Le Clerc, Haller, Sprengel, &c., or to some of those which relate especially to Hippo- crates, He divides the causes of disease into two principal classes ; the one comprehending the in- fluence of seasons, climates, water, situation, &c., and the other consisting of more personal and pri- vate causes, such as result from the particular kind and amount of food and exercise in which each separate individual indulges himself. The modifi- cations of the atmosphere dependent on different seasons and climates is a subject which was suc- cessfully treated by Hippocrates,

and which is still far from exhausted by all the researches of modern
science. He considered that while heat and cold, moisture and dryness,
succeeded one another throughout the year, the human body
underwent certain analogous changes, which influenced the diseases of
the period ; and on this basis was founded the doctrine of pathological
constitutions, corresponding to particular conditions of the atmosphere, so that, whenever the year or the season exhibited a special
character in which such or such a temperature prevailed, those persons
who were exposed to its influence were affected by a series of
disorders, all bearing the same stamp. (How plainly the same idea runs
through the Observaii- ones Medicae of Sydenham, our *English Hippocrates* " need not be pointed out to those who are at all familiar with
his works.) Tlie belief in the influence which different climates exercise
on the human frame follows naturally from the theory just mentioned ;
for, in fact, a climate may be con- sidered as nothing more than a
permanent season, whose effects may be expected to be more power-
ful, inasmuch as the cause is ever at work upon mankind. Accordingly,
Hippocrates attributes to climate both the conformation of the body
and the disposition of the mind — indeed, almost every thing ; and if
the Greeks were found to be hardy freemen, and the Asiatics
effeminate slaves, he accounts for the difference of their characters by
that of the climates in which they lived. With respect to the second
class of causes producing disease, he attributed all sorts of disorders to
a vicious system of diet, which, whether excessive or defective, he
considered to be equally injurious ; and in the same way' he supposed
that, when bo- dily exercise was either too much indulged in or entirely
neglected, the health was equally likely to suffer, thougli by different
forms of disease. Into all the minutiae of the " Humoral Pathology " (as
it was called), which kept its ground in FJurope as the prevailing
doctrine of all the medical sects for more than twenty centuries, it
would be out of place to enter here. It will be sufficient to remind the
reader that the four fluids or humours of the body (blood, phlegm,
yellow bile, and black bile) were supposed to be the primary seat of
disease ; that health was the result of the due combination (or crash) of
these, and that, when this crasis was disturbed, disease was the
consequence ; that, iu the course of a disorder that was proceeding fa-
vourably, these humours underwent a certain change in quality (or
coction), which was the sign of returning health, as preparing the way
for the expulsion of the morbid matter, or crisis; and that these crises

had a tendency to occur at certain stated periods, which were hence called " critical days." {Brit, and For. Med. Rev.)

The medical practice of Hippocrates was cautious and feeble, so much so, that he was in after times reproached with letting his patients die, by doing nothing to keep them alive. It consisted chiefly in watching tiie operations of nature, and pro- moting the critical evacuations mentioned above ; so that attention to diet and regimen was the principal and often the only remedy that he em- ployed. Several hundred substances have been enumerated which are used medicinally in different parts of the Hippocratic Collection ; of these, by far the greater portion belong to the vegetable kingdom, as it would be in vain to look for any traces of chemistry in these early writings. In surgery, he is the author of the frequently quoted maxim, that " what cannot be cured by medicines is cured by the knife ; and what cannot be cured by the knife is cured by fire." The anatomical knowledge displayed in different parts of the Hip- pocratic Collection is scanty and contradictory, so much so, that the discrepancies on this subject constitute an important criterion in deciding the genuineness of the different treatises.

With regard to the personal character of Hip- pocrates, though he says little or nothing expressly about himself, yet it is impossible to avoid drawing certain conclusions from the characteristic passages scattered through the pages of his writings. He was evidently a person who not only had had great experience, but who also knew how to turn it to the best account ; and the number of moral reflections and apophthegms that we meet with in his writings, some of which (as, for example, " Life is short, and Art is long ") have acquired a sort of proverbial notoriety, show him to have been a profound thinker. He appears to have felt the moral obligations and responsibilities of his profession, and often tries to impress upon his readers the duties of care and attention, and kind- ness towards the sick, saying that a physician's first and chief consideration ought to be the re- storing his patient to health. The style of the Hippocratic writings, which are in the Ionic dialect, is so concise as to be sometimes extremely ohscure ; though this charge, which is as old as the time of Galen, is often brought too indiscriminately against the whole collection, whereas it applies, in fact especially only to certain treatises, which seem to be merely a collection of notes, such as De IJu- moribiis, De Alimeido^ De Ojjlcina Medici,

&c. In those writings, which are universally allowed to be genuine, we do not find this excessive brevity, though even these are in general by no means easy. {Brit, and For. Med. Rev.)

Of the great number of books published on the subject of the Hippocratic Collection, only a very few of the most modern and most useful can be here enumerated ; a fuller list may be found in Choulant's Handb. der li'ucherkunde fur die Aeltere Medicin, or his Biblioth. Medico- 1 Hi- tor. ; or in Ackermann's Historia Literaria Ilijypo- crutis. Fiiesii Oeco7iomia Ilippocrads is a very copious and learned lexicon, published in fol. Francof. 1588, and Gene v. I(i62. Sprengel'B Apologie des Hippocr. und seiner Grundsatze (Leipz. 1789, 1792, 2 vols. 8vo.), contains, among other matter, a Gennan translation of some of tlie genuine treatises, with a valuable commentary. The treatise by Ermerins, De Hippocr. Doctrina a Prognostice oriunda (Lugd. Bat. 1832, 4to,), de- serves to be carefully studied ; as also does Link's dissertation, Ueher die Theorien in den Hippocra- tisclien Schriften^ nebst Bemerkungen uber die Echt- I/eit dieser ScJinflen^ in the * *Abhandlungen der* Berlin. Akadem.*' 1814, 1815. Gruner's Censura Lil)rorum Hippocraieorum qua veri a fulsis^ intcgri a supj)ositis segreganiur, Vratislav. 1772, 8vo., con- tains a useful account of the amount of evidence in favour of each treatise of the collection, though his conclusions are not always to be depended on. See al«o Houdart, Etudes Histor. et Crit. sur la Vie et kc Doctrine d' Hippocr. Paris, 183G, 8vo.; Petersen, Hippocr. Nomine quae circuiiiferuntur Scripta ad Temporis Raiiones dispos. Hamburg, 1839, 4to. ; Meixner, Neue Prnfung der Eehtlieit und Reiliefolge S'dmmtlicher Schriften Hippocr.^ Miinchen, 1836, 1837, 8vo. [W. A. G.]

www.ingramcontent.com/pod-product-compliance
Lightning Source LLC
Chambersburg PA
CBHW071516210326
41597CB00018B/2783